Extending Medicare Reimbursement in Clinical Trials

Committee on Routine Patient Care Costs in
Clinical Trials for Medicare Beneficiaries

Henry J. Aaron and Hellen Gelband, *Editors*

INSTITUTE OF MEDICINE

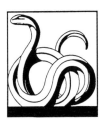

NATIONAL ACADEMY PRESS
Washington, D.C.

NATIONAL ACADEMY PRESS • 2101 Constitution Avenue, N.W. • Washington, DC 20418

NOTICE: The project that is the subject of this report was approved by the Governing Board of the National Research Council, whose members are drawn from the councils of the National Academy of Sciences, the National Academy of Engineering, and the Institute of Medicine. The members of the committee responsible for the report were chosen for their special competencies and with regard for appropriate balance.

Support for this project was provided by the Health Care Financing Administration (Contract No. 500-98-0275). The views presented in this report are those of the Institute of Medicine Committee on Routine Patient Care Costs in Clinical Trials for Medicare Beneficiaries and are not necessarily those of the funding agencies.

International Standard Book Number 0-309-06888-6

Additional copies of this report are available for sale from the National Academy Press, 2101 Constitution Avenue, N.W., Box 285, Washington, DC 20055. Call (800) 624-6242 or (202) 334-3313 (in the Washington metropolitan area), or visit the NAP online bookstore at **www.nap.edu**. The full text of this report is available on line at **www.nap.edu/readingroom**.

For more information about the Institute of Medicine, visit the IOM home page at **www.iom.edu**.

The serpent has been a symbol of long life, healing, and knowledge among almost all cultures and religions since the beginning of recorded history. The serpent adopted as a logotype by the Institute of Medicine is a relief carving from ancient Greece, now held by the Staatliche Museen in Berlin.

THE NATIONAL ACADEMIES

National Academy of Sciences
National Academy of Engineering
Institute of Medicine
National Research Council

The **National Academy of Sciences** is a private, nonprofit, self-perpetuating society of distinguished scholars engaged in scientific and engineering research, dedicated to the furtherance of science and technology and to their use for the general welfare. Upon the authority of the charter granted to it by the Congress in 1863, the Academy has a mandate that requires it to advise the federal government on scientific and technical matters. Dr. Bruce M. Alberts is president of the National Academy of Sciences.

The **National Academy of Engineering** was established in 1964, under the charter of the National Academy of Sciences, as a parallel organization of outstanding engineers. It is autonomous in its administration and in the selection of its members, sharing with the National Academy of Sciences the responsibility for advising the federal government. The National Academy of Engineering also sponsors engineering programs aimed at meeting national needs, encourages education and research, and recognizes the superior achievements of engineers. Dr. William A. Wulf is president of the National Academy of Engineering.

The **Institute of Medicine** was established in 1970 by the National Academy of Sciences to secure the services of eminent members of appropriate professions in the examination of policy matters pertaining to the health of the public. The Institute acts under the responsibility given to the National Academy of Sciences by its congressional charter to be an adviser to the federal government and, upon its own initiative, to identify issues of medical care, research, and education. Dr. Kenneth I. Shine is president of the Institute of Medicine.

The **National Research Council** was organized by the National Academy of Sciences in 1916 to associate the broad community of science and technology with the Academy's purposes of furthering knowledge and advising the federal government. Functioning in accordance with general policies determined by the Academy, the Council has become the principal operating agency of both the National Academy of Sciences and the National Academy of Engineering in providing services to the government, the public, and the scientific and engineering communities. The Council is administered jointly by both Academies and the Institute of Medicine. Dr. Bruce M. Alberts and Dr. William A. Wulf are chairman and vice chairman, respectively, of the National Research Council.

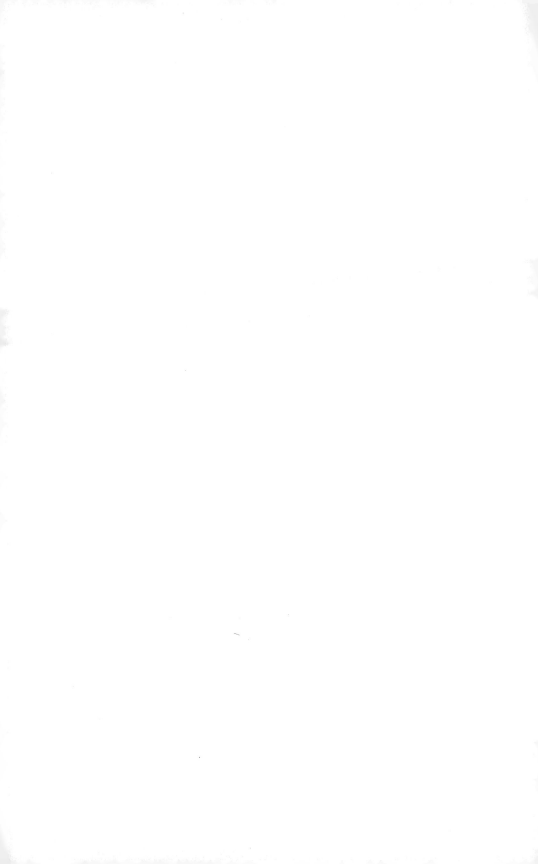

v

REVIEWERS

This report has been reviewed in draft form by individuals chosen for their diverse perspectives and technical expertise, in accordance with procedures approved by the National Research Council's Report Review Committee. The purpose of this independent review is to provide candid and critical comments that will assist the Institute of Medicine in making the published report as sound as possible and to ensure that the report meets institutional standards for objectivity, evidence, and responsiveness to the study charge. The review comments and draft manuscript remain confidential to protect the integrity of the deliberative process. The committee wishes to thank the following individuals for their participation in the review of this report:

HELEN L. SMITS, M.D., Ivoryton, Conn.
WADE AUBRY, M.D., The Lewin Group and University of California at San Franciooo
TOM AULT, Health Policy Alternatives, Washington, D.C.
PATRICIA A. BARR, J.D., Barr, Sternberg, and Moss, Bennington, Vt.
NORMAN DANIELS, Ph.D., Newton, Mass.
OLGA JONASSON, M.D., F.A.C.S., The American College of Surgeons, Chicago
ALAN S. LICHTER, M.D., University of Michigan Medical School
JAN PLATNER, J.D., JRI Health/Justice Resource Institute, Boston
ROBERT YOUNG, M.D., Fox Chase Cancer Center, Philadelphia

Although the individuals listed above have provided constructive comments and suggestions, it must be emphasized that responsibility for the final content of this report rests entirely with the authors and the Institute of Medicine.

Acknowledgments

We thank the following people for providing information or other assistance during the course of this project.

Wade Aubry	University of California at San Francisco
Grant P. Bagley	Health Care Financing Administration
Carmella Bocchino	American Association of Health Plans
Charles A. Coltman, Jr.	San Antonio Cancer Institute
Chuck Cutler	Prudential HealthCare
Ronald Herberman	Association of American Cancer Institutes
Doug Kamerow	Agency for Health Care Policy and Research
Deborah Kamin	American Society of Clinical Oncology
Allen S. Lichter	University of Michigan School of Medicine
Joanne R. Less	Food and Drug Administration
Sridhar Mani	Montefiore Medical Center, Albert Einstein College of Medicine
Mary McCabe	National Cancer Institute
Alexa McCray	National Library of Medicine
Charles J. McDonald	American Cancer Society
Stephen J. Northrup	Medical Device Manufacturers Association
Michael O'Connell	Mayo Clinic Cancer Center
Arnold Potosky	National Cancer Institute
Richard Rettig	Rand Corporation
Richard L. Schilsky	University of Chicago Cancer Research Center
Ellen M. Smith	General Accounting Office
Fran Visco	National Breast Cancer Coalition
Judith L. Wagner	Congressional Budget Office
Robert C. Young	Fox Chase Cancer Center

Contents

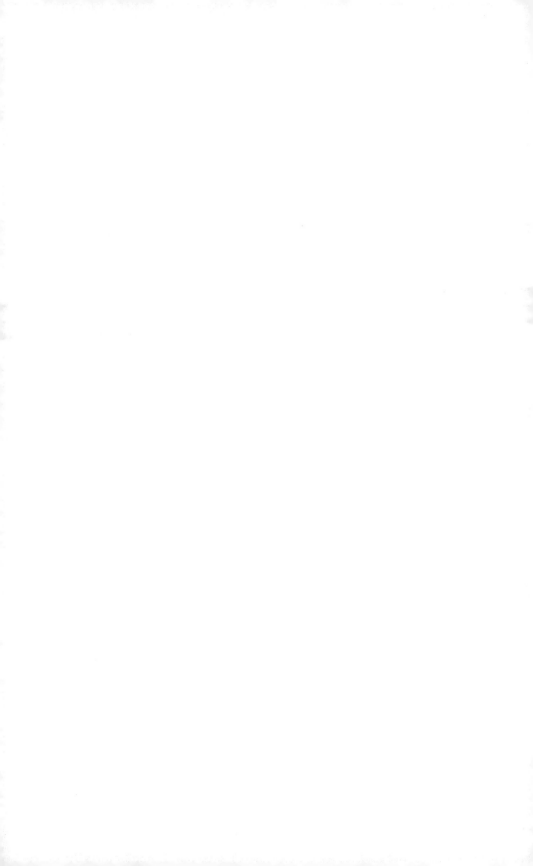

Executive Summary

BACKGROUND

Clinical trials have become an essential component of modern medical care. The breakneck speed of medical advances and the increased effort to base clinical decisions on reliable evidence place clinical trials in an ever more prominent position between medical innovation and medical practice. Expanding the evidence base for health care interventions is clearly in the interest of both taxpayers who support Medicare and beneficiaries who receive services.

The impression is widespread that some patient care in clinical trials is not reimbursable under Medicare. But except in the case of certain investigational medical devices and a few instances of "coverage with conditions," the Health Care Financing Administration (HCFA) has never explicitly laid out exactly what should and should not be reimbursed. This omission has led to varying interpretations of HCFA's intent by its fiscal intermediaries and carriers who process claims, as well as by providers submitting claims.

A large proportion of patient care provided in clinical trials is routine—care that would be eligible for reimbursement if delivered outside of a trial. Although the evidence is limited, it appears that claims for much of this care are submitted to HCFA (and other insurers, for non-Medicare patients) without acknowledgment that the patient is in a clinical trial, and they are paid in the normal course of business by HCFA's contractors. But not all such costs for clinical trial patients are paid.

Increasingly over the past five years, uncertainty about reimbursement for routine patient care has been suspected as contributing to problems enrolling people in clinical trials. Clinical trial investigators cannot guarantee that Medicare will pay for the care required, and they must disclose this uncertainty to potential participants during the informed consent process. Since Medicare does not routinely

1

"preauthorize" care (as do many commercial insurers) the uncertainty cannot be dispelled in advance. Thus, patients considering whether to enter trials must assume that they may have to pay bills that Medicare rejects simply because they have enrolled in the trial.

This report recommends an explicit policy for reimbursement of routine patient care costs in clinical trials. It further recommends that HCFA provide additional support for selected clinical trials, and that the government support the establishment of a national clinical trials registry. These policies (1) should assure that beneficiaries would not be denied coverage merely because they have volunteered to participate in a clinical trial; and (2) would not impose excessive administrative burdens on HCFA, its fiscal intermediaries and carriers, or investigators, providers, or participants in clinical trials. Explicit rules would have the added benefit of increasing the uniformity of reimbursement decisions made by Medicare fiscal intermediaries and carriers in different parts of the country. Greater uniformity would, in turn, decrease the uncertainty about reimbursement when providers and patients embark on a clinical trial.

CONTEXT OF THE CURRENT STUDY

In the Balanced Budget Act of 1997 (P.L. 105-33, Section 4108), Congress directed HCFA to enter into a contract with the National Academy of Sciences for a "Study on Preventive and Enhanced Benefits" under Medicare. Five specific items were to be studied:

1. nutrition therapy services, including parenteral and enteral nutrition and the provision of such services by a registered dietitian;
2. skin cancer screening;
3. medically necessary dental care;
4. *routine patient care costs for beneficiaries enrolled in approved clinical trial programs;*
5. elimination of time limitation for coverage of immunosuppressive drugs for transplant patients.

Three committees were established to carry out the tasks, including this one to focus exclusively on the clinical trial question.

The clinical trial committee is aware that the question of reimbursement for care in clinical trials is not a new issue. Clinical trial investigators, patients, and potential volunteers have increasingly seen as a problem the lack of coverage for routine patient care that would be covered if the patient were not in the trial. Cancer activists and organizations, including cancer centers, were the most active agents in bringing this issue into public view. Several draft bills have mandated that Medicare cover routine care costs in clinical trials. Some have named only "cancer trials," while others have pointed to "cancer and other life-threatening diseases." Agreements to pay for treatment in cancer trials have been drawn up between the National Cancer Institute (NCI) and the departments of Defense (DoD) and Veterans Affairs (VA); and United Healthcare, a major managed care organization, does pay for treatment (at varying levels) in selected cancer trials.

CLINICAL TRIALS

In this report, we define the term "clinical trial" as a formal study carried out according to a prospectively defined protocol. Clinical trials are intended to discover or verify the safety and effectiveness in human beings of interventions to promote well-being, or to prevent, diagnose, or treat illness. Other definitions are more expansive, including even the first use of a new intervention without a formal plan or any type of comparison. Our definition is limited to the activities that could be eligible for having at least some patient care costs reimbursed under Medicare. This definition includes:

- interventions to prevent, diagnose, and treat disease;
- drugs and devices; surgical, manipulative, and other procedures; diagnostic laboratory tests, scans, and examinations; dietary, behavioral, and psychological techniques;
- interventions associated with any illnesses or conditions (not limited to specific ones such as cancer, AIDS, and heart disease);
- new interventions, as well as "standard" interventions that have been used in a limited way (or extensively, but about which not enough reliable information is available).

This definition does not include a new intervention applied by a single practitioner to a single patient in what might be the earliest phase of innovation. It applies only after a protocol describing the intervention, the types of patients, the endpoints, and other details has been developed to find out whether an intervention is safe and effective for a given condition. For all types of interventions, the definition encompasses the comparative trials that are needed to produce definitive evidence, and for drugs and devices, in particular, the definition also includes early trials that may be focused mainly on safety and have only one intervention group ("single-arm trials," i.e., they do not compare outcomes in one group versus another; they simply observe what happens when the intervention is given).

The central importance of research to medical practice is relatively new. In the past, when few effective medical interventions were available and most cost relatively little, the lack of precise information about their effects made less difference to the public's health or wealth (although people were adversely affected by interventions that were not only ineffective but harmful). What is often cited as the first deliberately randomized clinical trial took place in the late 1940s to determine the efficacy of treating tuberculosis with a newly invented antibiotic, streptomycin. Over the years, occasional tragic complications associated with new drugs or devices led Congress to authorize regulatory agencies to mandate clinical trials to determine safety and efficacy before drugs and devices could be marketed in the United States. Although at least a minimal level of evidence from clinical trials is required for the legal marketing of drugs, biologics, and medical devices, information on whether a new drug or device works better than an old one is not required by law. And there is no such legal requirement to demonstrate safety or efficacy, to say nothing of superiority over existing procedures, for a new procedure that does not involve new commercial products. As a consequence, although many decisions are being made on the basis of sound evidence from clinical trials, the use of many medical interventions, old and new, does not rest on solid evidence. The new emphasis on evidence reflects the realization that intelligent decisions require substantial information that properly conducted clinical trials can provide.

CURRENT MEDICARE REIMBURSEMENT RULES RELATING TO INVESTIGATIONAL MEDICAL SERVICES AND CLINICAL TRIALS

The legislation establishing the Medicare program states:

> Notwithstanding any other provisions of this title, no payment may be made for items or services which are not reasonable and necessary for the diagnosis and treatment of illness or injury or to improve the functioning of a malformed body member.

Since the inception of the Medicare program in the mid-1960s, the phrase "reasonable and necessary" has guided Medicare reimbursement. Although little explicit policy has been issued on the topic, this clause has been the basis for excluding reimbursement for at least some routine patient care in clinical trials. This Medicare interpretation has historical roots in the private insurance sector, whose policies in the 1960s and still, in 1999, exclude coverage of services in clinical trials (GAO, 1999). Most private insurance plans have excluded coverage of services in clinical trials on the basis that the treatment is "experimental" or "investigational," although the language does not explicitly mention clinical trials (GAO, 1999).* However, Medical Directors report that they often approve

---

*The language regarding experimental and investigational treatment in most health insurance contracts is similar to the following, which is taken from a current Group Service Agreement of CIGNA Healthcare of New York, Inc.: "By way of example, but not limita-

payment for care in clinical trials on a case-by-case basis. In addition, private insurers have been involved in supporting specific trials (e.g., the Blue Cross/Blue Shield Association was instrumental in initiating a trial of high-dose chemotherapy with bone marrow transplant rescue for women with advanced breast cancer).

Despite the lack of an explicit Medicare policy excluding reimbursement for routine care in clinical trials, HCFA has signaled its intent in several ways in recent years. In 1993, HCFA asked the Office of the Inspector General (OIG) of the Department of Health and Human Services (DHHS) to investigate whether hospitals were billing Medicare "improperly for millions of dollars worth of surgical procedures involving unapproved medical devices," specifically investigational pacemakers, defibrillators, and other cardiac devices in clinical trials. In a 1996 hearing of the Subcommittee on Investigations of the Senate Committee on Governmental Affairs, an official of the OIG reported their finding that most of the 130 hospitals they investigated had, in fact, improperly billed Medicare for implanting investigational devices. The Inspector General urged HCFA to recover these "overpayments" from the hospitals (Hartwig, 1996).

What might not be clear from the OIG account is that it was not only payment for the investigational devices themselves, but for the implantation *procedures*, as illustrated by comments of others, including at least one HCFA official.*

---

tion, the following are specifically excluded services and benefits: "Medical, surgical or other health care procedures and treatments which are experimental or investigational, as determined by the HEALTHPLAN Medical Director in accordance with consensus derived from peer review medical and scientific literature and the practice of the national medical community, including (1) any procedures or treatments which are not recognized as conforming to accepted medical practice; (2) any procedures or treatments in which the scientific assessment of the technique, or its application for a particular condition, has not been completed or its effectiveness has not been established; and (3) any procedures or treatments for which the required approval of a government agency has not been granted at the time the services are rendered." GAO (1999) confirmed in interviews with health plan Medical Directors that this language is interpreted to exclude routine care in clinical trials. Most Medical Directors interviewed by GAO also stated that they make exceptions and do cover clinical trial costs on a case-by-case basis.

*This point was made clearly by a HCFA official testifying at the same hearing (Ault, 1996), who stated:

> Medicare's program instructions on medical devices, which were governing until November 1, 1995, were added to the Medicare Hospital Manual, the Carrier Manual, and the Intermediary Manual in 1986. These instructions stated clearly that "medical devices which have not been approved for marketing by the FDA are considered investigational by Medicare and are not reasonable and necessary." The instructions went on to explain that payment would not be made either for the devices or the procedures and services performed using the devices. Additional instructions in these manuals dealing more generally with

By the time of the hearing, HCFA had already changed its policy to allow reimbursement for patients in certain trials involving investigational devices (FDA "Category B" devices, which are refinements of, or very similar to, approved devices) but not for trials of other types of interventions. The clearest indication that routine patient care is not reimbursable in other types of trials is found in a 1997 report by the General Accounting Office (GAO, 1997) on reimbursement by HCFA for Medicare beneficiaries in cancer clinical trials. GAO found that reimbursement was, indeed, occurring without HCFA's knowledge. In responding to GAO's draft report, HCFA reported that their actuaries had "nearly doubled their estimates of the extent to which Medicare mistakenly reimburses claims for routine patient care costs. Under HCFA's current policy, any reimbursement for care associated with a cancer clinical trial would be made in error" (GAO, 1997).

HCFA has not issued any new language to change clinical trial reimbursement policy since the 1995 change for trials involving Category B medical devices, and no HCFA statements contradictory to what is presented here were found in the course of this study.

The 1995 agreement between HCFA and FDA constitutes the only formal statement of policy about reimbursement of routine patient care costs in clinical trials, authorizing reimbursement for those costs in most trials of investigational medical devices.

THE STATUS QUO IN REIMBURSEMENT

There is relatively little information about how the costs of patient care in clinical trials are actually paid, and the extent to which insurers are paying these costs, either knowingly or unknowingly. What information is available suggests that a sizable proportion is paid for by insurers, including HCFA. This conclusion derives from:

- direct evidence from one study that HCFA has paid unknowingly for most routine care of Medicare beneficiaries in certain cancer trials (GAO, 1997),
- evidence that, in the past (before the 1995 change in policy) HCFA unknowingly paid millions of dollars in reimbursement for Medicare beneficiaries in medical device trials (Hartwig, 1996),
- interviews with clinical trial investigators conducted for this study, in which they uniformly acknowledged submitting claims for reimbursement to HCFA and other insurers for routine patient care in trials and getting them paid,

---

all noncovered services also state that any services related to a noncovered service are excluded from coverage.

The official also made clear in his testimony that Medicare would have paid for patients in the trials to have the standard device implanted.

- interviews with private-sector clinical trial sponsors conducted for this study who stated that, while they do cover the costs of "protocol-induced" services, in general they do not provide money to pay for routine patient care; they expect providers to bill insurers for those costs,
- deduction, given the lack of another obvious source of payment for most routine care in trials, and
- lack of evidence from any source that HCFA and other insurers are *not* reimbursing for this care.

Providers violated no clear rules in billing for routine patient care costs in clinical trials because no such rules were ever codified. But the gap between the *impressions*—and statements of responsible HCFA officials—regarding reimbursement rules on the one hand, and reimbursement *practices* on the other hand, should be ended.

RECOMMENDATIONS

RECOMMENDATION 1. Medicare should reimburse routine care for patients in clinical trials in the same way it reimburses routine care for patients not in clinical trials.

This principle applies to payments for physicians and other providers, routine laboratory and other diagnostic tests, and any other services that comprise routine care for a given patient. All coverage and medical necessity rules and all other restrictions that apply to patients not in clinical trials would apply to care in clinical trials.

The committee recommends a broad definition of clinical trials—including all phases and legitimate designs and all sources of sponsorship (government, industry, or other)—all of which should be equally eligible for reimbursement. This definition does not mean, however, that any treatment simply called a "clinical trial" would qualify for reimbursement. To qualify, a clinical trial must have a written protocol that describes a scientifically sound study and have been approved by all relevant IRBs before participants are enrolled. HCFA should articulate criteria for an acceptable trial and IRB review, which investigators would apply to determine whether their studies are eligible for reimbursement. (HCFA could state the criteria in terms of "current NIH standards," e.g., rather than stating specific study characteristics.) The committee recognizes that controversies surround both the quality of current clinical trials and IRBs, but holds that these issues are being addressed in various ways by DHHS and other sectors of government, and should not be addressed routinely in HCFA's reimbursement decisions.

Medicare should reimburse *routine patient care* costs, but not *all* costs in clinical trials. Medicare should *not reimburse* the costs of experimental interventions (except category B devices for which reimbursement is allowed under agreement with FDA, and certain procedures as described in recommendation 2), of data collection and record keeping that would not be required but for the trial, or of other services to clinical trial participants necessary solely to satisfy data collection needs of the clinical trial ("protocol-induced costs"). These costs should remain the responsibility of research sponsors, private and public.

Medicare should continue its current practice of reimbursing costs of treating conditions that result as unintended consequences (complications) of clinical trials.

RECOMMENDATION 2. HCFA should reimburse surgeons (or other practitioners) for treating patients in randomized clinical trials involving procedures that are variations or modifications of accepted procedures, or new uses for accepted procedures.

Under the current interpretation of Medicare reimbursement rules, the committee believes that surgeons and others performing surgical or other procedures in trials might not be eligible to be reimbursed for those services. Therefore, the committee recommends that procedures that have become widely accepted as a part of standard medical practice, but which, as part of a clinical trial, are being rigorously evaluated, or are being modified or applied for new indications to determine the incremental risks and benefits, should be eligible for reimbursement at the rate for the standard procedure. Conversely, *types* of procedures for which initial questions of safety and efficacy have not been resolved would not be eligible for reimbursement.

Unlike the basic recommendation regarding routine patient care costs, which applies to *all* clinical trials, this recommendation would limit reimbursement to *randomized* trials (the equivalent of "phase 3" trials for drugs and devices). The committee believes this limitation is appropriate in order to avoid providing reimbursement for uncontrolled experimentation by practitioners. The introduction of new drugs and devices is governed by FDA under a formal system that involves phased trials. In contrast, the introduction of new procedures is not governed by any regulatory authority. In their early phases, procedures are modified or tried for different indications in clinical practice, but rarely in formal trials. However, once a new or modified procedure has been defined and developed to the point that it is distinct enough from the predicate procedure, it may be tested against the standard treatment (the predicate procedure or other accepted treatment) in a formal randomized trial. Medicare should provide reimbursement to the surgeon or other practitioner for treating patients in such trials.

Further clarification may be needed to make clear the committee's intent with regard to reimbursement for procedures on patients in clinical trials. The committee is expressing no judgments about when trials of procedures should or should not be carried out, or who should be involved in them if they are. This recommendation is not intended to influence the criteria or processes HCFA uses to decide on *coverage* of new procedures under usual medical care. It applies only when a trial of a procedure is being done—for all the reasons that trials are done—and claims for *reimbursement* for the procedure are submitted by practitioners.

HCFA's initial task in implementing this recommendation will be to develop definitions for classifying procedures analogous to "category A" and "category B" devices. These definitions describing what is and is not allowed will be applied in the field when claims are submitted. HCFA should *not* be required to rule routinely on the eligibility of procedures before bills may be submitted. In the same way that providers are responsible for following reimbursement rules for all services under Medicare, they will be responsible for applying the rules appropriately in the case of procedures in clinical trials. Fiscal intermediaries and carriers audit these interpretations by providers in clinical trials, as they now audit bills from providers who are not in clinical trials. Advice or an interpretation could, of course, be requested of HCFA at any time. In addition, HCFA would retain the right to initiate its own review, without being asked, if it believes there is an issue to be explored, to carry out a random check, or for another reason.

The committee recognizes that creating definitions that neatly separate "category A" and "category B" procedures will not be simple, and disagreements are inescapable about where the line between "A" and "B" should be drawn in specific cases.

Wherever the separation lies, some procedures will fall into a "gray zone." HCFA can narrow the gray zone by applying the definitions to a wide range of real and hypothetical procedures, and stating whether the procedures would or would not be eligible for reimbursement. To deal with cases in which uncertainty remains, HCFA should set up a process to rule quickly on reimbursement eligibility. With accumulated experience, the number of gray zone cases should decline, as has been the case with FDA classification of devices into categories A and B.

The committee has not attempted to specify an institutional mechanism under which HCFA might carry out the tasks required by this recommendation. However, the committee notes that the new Medicare Coverage Advisory Committee[*] might provide the needed expertise for the task of defining categories A and B and ruling quickly on "gray zone" cases that arise.

RECOMMENDATION 3. For claims submitted in accordance with both the fundamental recommendation (No. 1) and the special

---

[*]The Medicare Coverage Advisory Committee (MCAC) was established by HCFA to provide guidance on coverage issues. The 120-member committee will function through specialty panels of not more than 15 members each. The MCAC had its first meeting in September 1999.

recommendation for procedures (No. 2), no special precertification by HCFA, or any other administrative process, should be required of clinical trial researchers or providers participating in trials before they submit claims for covered services. Claims should be submitted in the same way they are for treatment outside of trials.

Practitioners and institutions would be expected to submit reimbursement claims for services to patients in clinical trials under rules outlined in Recommendations 1 and 2. With a clear statement of reimbursement policy, such claims should pose difficulties no different from those arising in the administration of coverage and reimbursement rules for claims for care outside of trials.

Investigators and providers would not be routinely required to submit documentation about the trial to HCFA, but HCFA could, at any time, request such documentation to confirm that the clinical trial meets current standards for scientific merit and has the relevant IRB approval.

RECOMMENDATION 4. If Medicare or trial sponsors fail to cover clinical care costs, patients should not be billed for those costs above what they would pay if they were not in a trial.

This recommendation is not one that can be enforced as part of a reimbursement policy by HCFA; however, the committee believes it is an important principle that could be adopted by clinical trial sponsors and investigators. It also could be incorporated in any legislation passed to implement the committee's recommendations.

RECOMMENDATION 5. Medicare members of managed care plans should have the same reimbursement eligibility for care in clinical trials as those enrolled in fee-for-service Medicare, but not beyond the limits of the managed care contract.

Nearly one Medicare beneficiary in five belongs to a capitated plan—an HMO or some other form of managed care. That number is likely to increase over time. It is vital, therefore, that the committee's recommendations carry over to patients served outside traditional Medicare. Managed care plans must provide all benefits offered under traditional Medicare. (Most offer additional benefits, including coverage of outpatient drugs.) Accordingly, the committee recommends that managed care plans be required to offer Medicare beneficiaries access to clinical trials involving services available within their networks. If, for example, a plan routinely covers a particular drug, it should cover it in a trial, as well. If the plan limits the choice of drugs to those listed on a formulary, the plan should not be required to cover a nonformulary drug in a trial.

Under point-of-service plans, patients should have the right to go outside the managed care network to participate in a trial, under the terms stipulated in the plan for point-of-service care, but no such right should be inferred under plans that limit enrollees to the plan's providers. This recommendation is not comprehensive, but is suggestive of a policy for managed care. Full implementation will require additional thought when HCFA adopts a clinical trial reimbursement policy, but the committee urges that the new policy not create obstacles to clinical trial enrollment for beneficiaries in managed care.

RECOMMENDATION 6. In addition to providing routine coverage through the proposed policy, the committee urges HCFA to use its existing authority to support selected trials and to assist in the development of new trials. In selected clinical trials, the committee believes that HCFA should do more than pay for routine patient care according to the recommendations already stated. Medicare should (1) provide additional reimbursement in a limited number of trials and (2) identify emerging or current methods of care of particular importance to the Medicare population and work with other organizations to initiate trials.

Researchers should be able to apply to HCFA for reimbursement above routine rates in cases meriting special treatment. Such trials could include some interventions that do not qualify under the basic recommendations, such as "category A" procedures, primary and secondary screening, diagnostics, and interventions not usually covered by Medicare (e.g., behavioral interventions). The rationale for extending coverage is straightforward. HCFA has a large stake in determining whether more effective or less costly alternatives to current interventions may exist, preventing ineffective procedures from becoming common practice, and facilitating the identification of innovations that would benefit the Medicare population.

For example, a behavioral intervention, which normally would not be covered, might replace a more expensive drug or surgical intervention to the benefit of both patients' health and Medicare finances. HCFA should have sole authority to decide whether to extend coverage and should make such determinations expeditiously. The committee assumes that only a few trials would be appropriate for such exceptional treatment each year.

In the case of interventions of particular importance to the Medicare population, HCFA should collaborate with the National Institutes of Health (NIH) or others to see that appropriate trials are fielded. HCFA should cover routine patient care costs for these trials along the lines of the committee's basic recommendation. It could also fund other costs as well, under the exceptions procedure described in the preceding paragraph. But the objective is to encourage trials, not necessarily to pay for them. Such an active role would not be new for HCFA. This recommendation follows the model of the ongoing study of lung volume reduction surgery, which grew out of collaboration among HCFA, NIH, and the Agency for Health Care Policy and Research (AHCPR), at HCFA's initiative.

> **RECOMMENDATION 7. Every trial for which some Medicare reimbursement is sought should be entered into a national registry of clinical trials.**

Reimbursement claims should bear an identification number assigned by the registry. A registry will facilitate *ex post* audits of reimbursement claims, HCFA's main tool for monitoring clinical trial coverage and detecting potential abuse. But identification of a claim as part of a clinical trial should not be relevant to the reimbursement decision.

The committee recognizes that implementation of this recommendation will necessarily take some time. Therefore, the committee's recommendations regarding reimbursement of routine patient care costs do not hinge on the existence of a clinical trials registry. Until a registry is in operation, reimbursement claims for interventions associated with a clinical trial should be denoted on the form, in a manner HCFA specifies. However, a registry would contribute to uniform administration and permit HCFA and others to carry out analyses of clinical trials and the costs of implementing the recommendations put forward here. It should, therefore, be put in place as quickly as possible.

Ideally, such a registry should include all publicly and privately sponsored trials before they begin accruing patients, thereby providing a link to all claims for Medicare patients in clinical trials. If the goal of creating such a registry is accepted, the practical question of how best to achieve it must be addressed. It would be possible to build upon the registry currently under development at NIH by broadening the definition of trials to be included and consulting widely on how to present data. Or a separate registry could be created.

Whether the registry should operate within NIH or elsewhere merits consideration. The design of the NIH registry has been underway for some time. Its designers claim that it will be functioning, at least in part, by early 2000. Redirecting any ongoing effort will be difficult for reasons that are well understood. If it were concluded that converting this limited registry into an inclusive national registry would be needlessly cumbersome, the creation of a separate comprehensive registry, serving objectives beyond those of NIH, or even of HCFA, should be explored. The committee urges the Secretary of DHHS to examine this issue promptly, set a timetable for completion of a registry, and seek adequate funding for it.

ADMINISTRATIVE AND COST IMPLICATIONS

Implementation of the committee's recommendations would likely cause some increase in administrative costs to HCFA. In making its recommendations, the committee strove to minimize potential administrative burdens. It is the committee's assertion that any added administrative costs required by institution of this reimbursement policy will be small.

Effects of the committee's recommendations on benefit costs are more important and far more uncertain. For several reasons, the cost impact of these recommendations is likely to be quite small. First, the recommended reimbursement policy is designed to limit payments for an individual to roughly the cost of "standard care" for which he or she would be eligible if not enrolled in the trial. This limitation does not imply that each individual would have chosen standard care that cost the same as the care in the clinical trial, so in individual cases, the cost of actual care in the trial might be higher or lower than forgone care outside the trial. Although the incremental cost of routine care in clinical trials is not known with certainty, it is almost surely small in comparison to the costs otherwise incurred by Medicare. Some clinical trial groups claim that the costs of treating patients in some trials may be less than treating them outside of trials. Second, clinical trials hold the long-term prospect of identifying ineffective interventions, which would fall out of favor in the clinical community, or could be excluded from coverage, in some cases saving Medicare dollars.

Finally, only a tiny fraction of Medicare patients participate in clinical trials. No accurate count of clinical trial participants at any point in time exists, but the Lewin Group has estimated that about 265,000 people in the United States participate in clinical trials each year, including about 161,000 Medicare beneficiaries—less than 0.5 percent of the 38 million Medicare enrollees in 1997 (Dobson and Sturm, 1999). Clearly, the proportion of Medicare beneficiaries in clinical trials is quite small. The available evidence suggests that Medicare already pays 50 to 90 percent of routine patient care in such trials. These estimates take into account both costs for which no reimbursement is sought, and claims that are submitted and rejected.

The largest effect on Medicare costs could come from the speedier determination of the efficacy of innovative or experimental procedures, drugs, and devices. Some will be cost increasing. Others will be cost reducing. Whether the net effect is to raise or lower total Medicare spending, the speedy determination of what works and what does not work will benefit the Medicare population and the nation as a whole.

CONCLUSION

Clinical trials are integral to modern medical care and to the progress of medical science. Although HCFA has issued little explicit policy about payment for routine care for patients in clinical trials, the Medicare statute has been widely interpreted to exclude reimbursement for such care. However, evidence is ample to suggest that providers submit claims for routine care for Medicare beneficiaries in trials without noting the existence of the clinical trial, and HCFA's financial contractors usually pay them. The thrust of the committee's recommendations is that nothing should be done that would materially curtail Medicare's reimbursement for routine patient care costs for patients in clinical trials. On the contrary, HCFA should encourage such trials and even extend reimbursement in a limited number of specifically approved exceptional cases. To achieve these goals, the committee believes that HCFA should assure patients in clinical trials the same reimbursement of routine patient care that is available to patients who are not in trials. Extending reimbursment to certain procedures that represent modifications of current practice and distinguishing those from procedures for which risks and benefits are largely unknown will require some additional effort by HCFA, but it is an essential component of the committee's recommendations. The fundamental recommendation—reimbursement independent of trial participation—should be implemented relatively easily.

1

Clinical Trials in the United States

BACKGROUND ON CLINICAL TRIALS

A clinical trial is a formal study carried out according to a prospectively defined protocol. It is intended to discover or verify the safety and effectiveness in human beings of interventions to promote well-being, or to prevent, diagnose, or treat illness. Other definitions are more expansive—including even the first use of a new intervention in a human being, without a formal plan or any type of comparison—or more restrictive—including only studies comparing two or more interventions concurrently.

Properly conducted clinical trials are a necessity in health care because very few interventions produce such large or striking results that they can be evaluated by observation alone. Most often, the effects of an intervention are modest, perhaps a reduction of 10 percent in the risk of an important outcome. Such effects can be extremely important, however, especially when the endpoint is death from some common disease that kills thousands (or tens of thousands) of people each year. Differences of this magnitude cannot be detected reliably against the background of chance and other influences without a carefully planned and controlled study (Hennekens and Buring, 1987).

The common image of a clinical trial is the comparison of two (or more) interventions—new versus old (or versus placebo)—to see which one works better. Such trials are, in fact, relied upon to produce sound evidence for rational decision making in health care. To generate the most reliable information, clinical trials require certain design characteristics (particularly assignment of participants to interventions by "randomization"), and they must include enough participants to exclude the play of chance as a likely explanation for results. Regardless of the sophistication and complexity of the design and analysis, the question of whether "a" is better than "b" is the essence of the clinical trial. The interventions that might be tested go beyond treatments (pharmaceutical, biologic, radiologic, surgical, or other procedures) to include preventive strategies,

15

diagnostic tests, screening procedures, devices, and other forms of medical advice or patient care.

The definition of clinical trial used in this report encompasses some studies involving only a single intervention group. Such studies are included because they are often carried out before the definitive, comparative study to gather specific pieces of information about the intervention before the comparative study can proceed. To a great extent, these "single-arm," early phase clinical trials have been defined by the regulations governing approval of new drugs and are also a prominent feature of trials in cancer treatment (see Table 1-1). Their value lies in setting the stage for definitive, randomized trials. The committee believes that at least some patient care costs incurred in these trials should be eligible for Medicare reimbursement.

TABLE 1-1. Phases of Clinical Trials (usually applied to drugs and devices)

Phase 1	First studies in people, to evaluate chemical action, appropriate dosage, and safety. Usually enrolls small numbers of participants and typically has no comparison group.
Phase 2	Provides preliminary information about how well the new drug works and generates more information about safety and benefit. Usually includes comparison group; patients may be assigned to groups by randomization.
Phase 3	Compares intervention with the current standard or placebo to assess dosage effects, effectiveness, and safety. Almost always uses random allocation to assign treatment. Typically involves many people (hundreds or thousands) but may be smaller.
Phase 4	"Post-marketing surveillance," evaluates long-term safety (and sometimes effectiveness) for a given indication, usually after approval for marketing has been granted by FDA.

Brief History of Clinical Trials

The formal evolution of the clinical trial dates from the eighteenth century, but the concept of comparing how well people fare after being "assigned" to different "interventions" (e.g., diets or medical treatments) has ancient historical origins. A considerable body of literature traces major developments along the way. (e.g., Bull, 1959; Lilienfeld, 1982; Meinert, 1986).

The practice of randomization—randomly assigning study participants to either an experimental or a control group—was introduced by the statistician Ronald Fisher in horticultural research in 1926 and was described in his 1935 book (Fisher, 1926, 1935). Fisher asked the elemental question: How does one determine whether an observed difference in yield between fields is due to the difference in the seed or fertilizer being tested, or due to differences in soil, temperature, moisture, and light? Fisher proposed dividing plots of land into narrow strips and assigning experimental treatments their place in the soil by a chance mechanism. He pointed out that "randomization relieves the experimenter from the anxiety of considering and estimating the magnitude of the innumerable causes by which his data may be disturbed" (Fisher, 1935).

The British medical statistician Sir Austin Bradford Hill discussed the procedures of treatment allocation in 1937 (Doll, 1982), but time elapsed before medical researchers recognized that Fisher's ideas had applications beyond the bounds of farming research. Hill and the British Medical Research Council, in their multicenter trial of streptomycin in patients with tuberculosis (Medical Research Council, 1948), are recognized as the first to use random sampling numbers to allocate patients to experimental and control groups. This trial also set standards for modern trials by defining, in advance, the characteristics of patients who would and would not be admitted to the trial; objectively documenting the response to treatment; and establishing a neutral committee to deliberate on the ethical concerns posed by the trial (e.g., whether it was ethical to withhold the drug from the control series, whether the physicians supervising the trial could modify the treatment schedule, and whether control patients should be given placebos that would permit the trial to be conducted in a double-blind manner).

It is only in the past few decades that the randomized controlled trial has emerged as the preferred method—"the gold standard"—for evaluating medical interventions. But in that span, approximately a quarter of a million reports of "controlled trials" (though not all randomized) have been carried out (Cochrane Library Controlled Trials Register,1999).

Characteristics of Current-Day Clinical Trials

Innovation is occurring continually in the design, conduct, and analysis of clinical trials, but most trials follow certain patterns and conventions. First (except for single-arm trials, discussed later in this chapter), they are comparative: two or more interventions are compared for efficacy or effectiveness.[*] The comparison is often between a new intervention and the current standard of care, which may be a completely different intervention, a placebo, no treatment, or the same intervention at a different dose or regimen or intensity. Trials also may

---

[*]Efficacy is defined as the extent to which an intervention produces a beneficial result under ideal conditions. Effectiveness is used to describe the extent to which a specific intervention, when used under ordinary circumstances, does what it is intended to do. Effectiveness, therefore, takes into account the fact that, in any group of individuals, some will not take the intervention as prescribed, or will take other actions that may compromise the effect of the intervention (e.g., take drugs that might interact with the test intervention). In this report, the recommendations apply to trials testing either efficacy or effectiveness.

compare two or more "standard" interventions, all of which may be effective to some extent, to find out which works best.

Participant Population and Sample Size

It is generally accepted that the types and numbers of participants to be sought for a trial must be determined before the trial can begin. The study population should clearly be related to the condition under study, for example, a new treatment for Alzheimer's disease should be tested on Alzheimer's patients. But should the population be restricted further to include only a certain age range or exclude specific other diseases that patients might have? An area of ongoing debate concerns whether a trial is strengthened by patients being more homogeneous or more heterogeneous (see, e.g., Zelen, 1993). In trials of screening technologies, for example, the population may be of "average risk" or may be at higher-than-average risk due to some known characteristics (e.g., family history of the screened condition).

The definition of participant characteristics directly affects how many participants need to be enrolled to answer the question addressed by the trial and how long the trial should be continued, which in turn affects the administrative structure needed to carry out the trial. The point of doing a randomized trial is to get a reliable answer, which requires avoiding undue influence of the play of chance, and this requires that sufficient numbers of "events" occur during the trial for chance to be ruled out as a likely explanation for the results. It is the number of "events"—that is, the number of participants who experience the outcome of interest during the course of the study—that drives the sample size and only indirectly the number of study participants. For instance, consider a hypothetical example of testing a yearlong intervention (e.g., an exercise program, or a drug) to prevent hip fractures. Enrolling people under age 40 would require far more people than would the same trial in people over age 70 because so few would be expected to experience hip fractures in the absence of the intervention. The trial of under 40s could also be done with the same numbers, but it would require several decades longer than the trial of over 70s. Real trade-offs must be made in reaching these decisions. In the example given here, perhaps the intervention has greater potential when begun at a young age, so the effect could be at least quantitatively (if not qualitatively) different than if only applied at an older age. The complexity and expense of carrying out the trial in the younger group might overwhelm any resources available (not to mention the fact that the technology might be obsolete by the time the decades-long study is complete), leaving researchers with little choice but to enroll older individuals.

Randomization and Blinding

It is widely accepted that participants must be assigned to intervention groups through randomization, a process that ensures an equal probability of getting any one of the treatments. Variations on the simplest form of the randomization process (a list of random numbers) have been developed to improve the balance of prognostic factors among intervention groups (e.g., stratification of participants before random assignment by potentially prognostic factors such as age, gender, or other medical conditions). However, the aim of the various methods is essentially the same.

Another important aspect of trial design is "blinding" (or "masking")—keeping secret which intervention each patient is getting—which may be built in at several levels. The purpose of blinding is to avoid any bias—conscious or unconscious—in interpreting the effects of the interventions. In many cases, it is possible to keep the patient and the practitioner blind to which intervention the participant is receiving. This is common in pharmaceutical trials, in which dummy pills, injections, or other products can be manufactured so that all the treatments appear to be the same to doctor and participant. Blinding is often more difficult for procedures. Surgeons and others carrying out procedures must know what they are, but it may be possible to keep the patient unaware. Even when the practitioner knows which participants received which intervention, outcomes can often be evaluated by a third party without that knowledge.

Baseline Characteristics and Outcomes

In clinical trials, participants are generally followed from a well-defined point (e.g., diagnosis), which becomes time zero, or baseline, for the study. Usually, baseline information is recorded for each participant. This information may be as basic as age and gender, or it may include the results of diagnostic tests such as imaging, endoscopy, biopsy, cytology, or laboratory tests. The distribution of these characteristics in the different intervention groups is used as one measure of assurance that the groups are similar. The assumption is that, with a large enough number of people randomized, both the known and unknown factors that may affect outcome will be approximately equally distributed.

The outcome measures may consist of laboratory test results, death or survival, a nonfatal clinical event, patients' symptoms or views, signs of disease, or quality of life. There may be various short- and long-term outcomes in a given trial, which are monitored in different ways. In a trial treating people just after a heart attack, short-term survival (e.g., one day, one week, one month) is the immediate goal, and that information can be recorded quickly in the hospital. Longer-term survival is also important, however, and tools exist in the United States (e.g., the National Death Index) and other countries through which the fact and cause of a person's death can be determined without directly contacting next-of-kin.

Analysis

The fundamental analysis of a controlled clinical trial is a comparison of the rates of important outcomes among the intervention groups. The difficult part is assuring that differences are due mainly to the different treatments, and not to chance or bias. The effect of chance is minimized by making the trial large enough, and the effect of bias is minimized by randomization, blinding, and other design features.

A key concept in analysis is that the fundamental comparison is between the entire group randomized to one intervention and the entire group randomized to another intervention *regardless of whether everyone in the groups actually got the intervention they were assigned.* This may seem counterintuitive, but the "intention-to-treat" analysis is the only unbiased method for comparing the interventions. This makes it important to try to get as many people as possible to partake of their assigned intervention, and to maintain complete follow up of participants

Trial Organization

Clinical trials are simple conceptually, but they involve large numbers of people and require a significant infrastructure to carry out properly. In order to complete a study in a reasonable period of time, it is common to enroll participants in several different sites (in some cases hundreds) in the United States or around the world, in "multicenter" trials. One site acts as a coordinating center, usually controlling randomization of patients at all centers. That center or another may contain a central laboratory, receiving thousands of aliquots of blood or other biological samples to analyze from all centers.

A critical component of a trial organization, particularly for larger randomized trials, is a "data safety and monitoring committee," which is independent of the trial investigators themselves. This committee's main responsibility is to the study participants. By conducting periodic reviews of interim data, they can determine whether, on one hand, any of the treatments have demonstrated a definitive benefit, or on the other, whether any of the interventions are clearly harmful. In either case, they have the authority to stop recruitment (and treatment, if it is appropriate) or modify the trial. Because of the complexity involved, there are no universal rules for deciding when a trial should be stopped.

Protecting the Rights of Trial Participants

Individuals joining clinical trials do not forfeit their individual rights to participate in their own health care decisions or to change their minds at any time, but they also may be limited in their ability to fully exercise these rights. Participants often are ill, which is why they are entering the trial, and are therefore vulnerable in decisions relating to their health. In addition, they may not understand all the intricacies of the trial or their alternatives. For these reasons, considerable effort has been put into instituting mechanisms that seek to assure the rights of participants in clinical trials.

The first line of protection comes from the trial protocol itself developed by the study investigators and approved by the data and safety monitoring committee (see *Trial Organization*, above). The protocol is a formal written document that describes the rationale for the trial, interventions, and other medical services that participants will get, numbers of participants needed, outcomes that will be measured, plan for analysis, and other details of the trial organization. The protocol is used to develop a patient consent form that describes the protocol, the potential benefits and risks, and the patients' rights in the trial, in nontechnical language. The information on the consent form, as well as information supplied by study investigators or other health care providers involved in the trial, forms the basis of "informed consent," which must be given by individuals before they can formally enroll in a trial. The aim of informed consent is to ensure that participants understand the potential benefits and risks of participating, as well as their rights during the trial.

The informed consent process and documentation follow detailed rules set out by the institutional review boards (IRBs) at each site where participants are enrolled. For trials funded by the federal government and trials involving medical interventions subject to federal regulation, these rules are dictated by the Department of Health and Human Services (DHHS) Regulations for the Protection of Human Subjects in the Code of Federal Regulations (45 C.F.R. §46). The Office for Protection from Research Risks (OPRR) in DHHS is the center for implementing the regulations and providing guidance on ethical issues in biomedical or behavioral research. All responsible host institutions require equivalent procedures, regardless of who is sponsoring the trial.

IRBs are charged with protecting human volunteers in biomedical research. This involves not only ensuring informed consent, but also all aspects of the trial that bear on the welfare of the participants. Before a trial can begin, each IRB reviews the protocol, including such aspects as existing knowledge relative to the arms of study, the participant population and recruitment, potential risks and benefits to participants and society, investigator credentials, and monitoring requirements for the trial. During the trial, the IRB receives regular, periodic reports from the investigators, which it reviews and discusses. The IRB has authority to stop recruitment or take other actions necessary to protect participants.

Interpreting Evidence from Clinical Trials

It is rare that a single clinical trial answers a question definitively. Commonly, many trials with modest numbers of participants are carried out, asking the same or related questions, with identical, similar, or loosely related interventions being tested. The challenge for decision makers (at all levels in health care, from central policy makers to the physician in the clinic) is to use all the reliable information available to determine the best intervention for a specific condition.

Specific techniques can be used to express the results from multiple clinical trials in single numbers, variously called "meta-analyses" or statistical "overviews." In their most detailed form, they use the original data for each participant randomized in each trial; other techniques use only published results to estimate an average result. The increasing reliance on meta-analyses has emphasized the need to have access to all the evidence from all the trials of a particular question—not only the trials with published results, and not only those funded by certain sponsors. The reason is that trials that are published differ from those that are not. "Publication bias" occurs for various reasons: researchers may be less likely to seek publication for a trial that has negative results (e.g., a new treatment was no better than an old one), journals may be less likely to accept trials with negative results, or trials funded by the pharmaceutical industry that do not support a product may be withheld from publication. Follow-up of "cohorts of initiated trials" confirms that those trials with positive findings are more likely to be published than those with negative findings (Dickersin and Min 1993). The impact on the evidence is clear: interventions that may, on balance, be ineffective or even harmful may be adopted because the published evidence is supportive while the negative evidence is unavailable.

The idea of "prospective registration" of clinical trials has been proposed as a way to diminish the problems caused by publication bias. Researchers looking into specific areas could search trials registries to find out what trials have been done or are under way and whether or not their results have been published. Results of unpublished trials could be sought out, if desired.

The topic of clinical trial registration is important to this report because one of the committee's recommendations requires linking Medicare claims for care received in the context of a clinical trial to a national clinical trials registry. An ongoing effort to establish such a registry is described at the end of this chapter.

SPONSORSHIP OF CLINICAL TRIALS

The federal government and the drug, biologic, and device industries sponsor most clinical trials in the United States. Private grant-making organizations and medical centers support small numbers of trials. Within the government, the National Institutes of Health (NIH) is the largest trial sponsor by far, but the Department of Veterans Affairs (VA) and the Department of Defense (DoD) also fund many. In addition, DHHS sponsors a few outside of NIH, through the Centers for Disease Control and Prevention (CDC) and the Agency for Health Care Policy and Research (AHCPR). Pharmaceutical and device companies mount clinical trials as a routine and necessary part of the process of securing federal approval for new products and adding approved indications to the labeling of existing products. Trials of new procedures (e.g., surgery or radiologic procedures) do not involve the approval of commercial products and are typically funded by NIH or a medical center where the trial is undertaken.

Clinical trials take place in a variety of settings, including academic and other medical centers, such as comprehensive cancer centers. In attempts to expand enrollment in trials and involve more practitioners, NIH has extended clinical trial networks to include community hospitals and other community-based providers in their trials. Trials sponsored by VA take place within VA facilities and associated medical centers. DoD-sponsored trials are mounted mostly at DoD facilities, and a small number take place in other settings. Trials sponsored by the government are usually managed by a team of academically affiliated investigators at a "coordinating center."

Industry sponsors trials at the same medical centers that run government-funded trials and collaborates directly with VA and other government entities. Industry also recruits private clinics and individual practitioners to enroll patients in trials. Companies run some trials directly, but more often they retain one of the growing number of "contract research organizations." These organizations, like the coordinating centers mentioned above, manage the day-to-day activities of trials, including recruiting collaborators, analyzing data, and writing reports.

Exactly how many clinical trials are under way in the United States is unknown, as is the number of people participating in them, but information is available for some categories. Some, but not all, NIH institutes have developed centralized lists of trials. Since the approval of an IRB is typically necessary to conduct trials, their existence is not confidential, but there is no easy way to find them all. Within the government, the Food and Drug Administration (FDA) has information about industry-funded trials for new drug and device applications, but FDA is bound to maintain the confidentiality of that information unless the sponsor chooses to make it public.

NIH-Sponsored Trials

Most NIH-sponsored trials are carried out under grants and contracts by researchers at universities, specialized treatment centers, and other medical settings. Some (particularly smaller phase 1 and 2) trials are conducted at the NIH Clinical Center in Bethesda, Maryland, by researchers employed by NIH.

Only a few NIH institutes maintain registries or lists of the trials they are currently sponsoring. Lists of trials in cancer, AIDS, eye conditions, and rare diseases are available. Overall, NIH estimates that it sponsors about 7,000 clinical research studies at any one time—including both clinical trials and more basic studies—but NIH does not estimate how many of these are clinical trials (McCray, 1999).

In 1999, NIH is sponsoring about 1,100 cancer treatment trials (about 400 are phase 3 randomized trials) and some smaller numbers of other trials (e.g., about 200 AIDS treatment trials and fewer than 100 trials in eye disease). NIH has estimated that about 108,000 individuals enter into NIH-sponsored clinical treatment trials (this excludes trials of disease prevention) each year, with the largest number (an estimated 30,000) in cancer treatment trials (O'Rourke, 1999).

Other Government-Sponsored Clinical Trials

VA has a long-standing "Cooperative Studies Program," through which it sponsors multicenter clinical trials of particular importance to veterans. About 60 such studies, most carried out over about a 5-year period, are under way (Department of Veterans Affairs, 1999). In addition, VA researchers collaborate with academic medical centers, NIH researchers, and private industry in conducting trials at VA sites. The majority of participants in VA trials are veterans eligible for health care through VA.

DoD sponsors some clinical trials for people in the uniformed services and their dependents. In recent years, Congress has allocated funds for special DoD research programs on breast cancer, prostate cancer, and ovarian cancer, and a small amount of these funds has gone toward funding clinical trials outside the DoD system.

Industry-Sponsored Clinical Trials

For the pharmaceutical, biotechnology, and device industries, clinical trials are part of the process of developing the necessary evidence of efficacy and safety for bringing new products to market. For the most part, the trials these companies conduct are prescribed by the laws and regulations governing approval of new products, under the regulatory authority of FDA. Companies may also conduct trials that involve only approved products, and some of these do not require notifying FDA.

CLINICAL TRIAL PROTOCOL REVIEW AND MONITORING

Clinical trials sponsored by the federal government undergo review before they are funded and allowed to proceed. The review consists of both examination of procedures by an IRB to ensure the rights and protections of participants, and some type of "peer" evaluation of the scientific design and technical aspects of the study (scientific and technical review also considers risks to human subjects). Although each sponsor develops scientific evaluation criteria independently, they are all similar. DHHS Regulations for the Protection of Human Subjects in the Code of Federal Regulations (45 CFR 46) establish standards for human subjects' protection in all clinical research funded by DHHS. OPRR implements the regulations and provides guidance on ethical issues in biomedical and behavioral research.

FDA does not conduct clinical trials, but it has a major review function. Clinical trials using pharmaceuticals, biologics, or devices not yet approved by FDA always requires that research protocols be filed with FDA. In some (but not all) cases, protocols filed with FDA are also required when already-approved drugs are being used experimentally in patient groups or in ways that are substantially different from those for which the drug was approved. These rules apply to all sponsors, government or private. FDA's authority derives from the Federal Food, Drug, and Cosmetic Act and is codified in Title 21 of the Code of Federal Regulations. All research undertaken under this authority also must adhere to the applicable federal regulations regarding the protection of human subjects.

COSTS OF PATIENT CARE IN CLINICAL TRIALS

Only evidence from pilot studies exists comparing the relative cost of patient care in clinical trials with the cost of treating similar patients in nonexperimental settings. These pilot studies were sponsored by the National Cancer Institute (NCI) in preparation for larger projects. Together, the studies compared the costs for about 260 patients in NCI-sponsored phase 2 and 3 cancer clinical trials with the costs of care for patients with similar diseases treated in the same health systems (Mayo Clinic, Group Health of Puget Sound, Kaiser Permanente of Northern California). Data from similar studies of patients in cancer trials have been presented at briefings and meetings, but written versions have not been available, and the methodology has not been described as thoroughly as it has for the three NCI-supported studies. Results from a larger NCI-funded study by the RAND Corporation should be available in a few years, but that study will also be limited to analyzing costs in NCI-funded cancer trials, excluding industry-funded trials. No studies of the costs of treating patients with other medical conditions in clinical trials are known to exist.

The NCI-Funded Pilot Studies[*]

All three studies relied on information from health system computerized databases, augmented by chart review. Efforts were made to match patients participating in clinical trials to patients receiving standard community care who were similar in all relevant respects and who would have been eligible to participate in the respective trial.

---

[*]This section is adapted from a summary prepared by Martin Brown (Applied Research Branch, National Cancer Institute), based on preliminary results of the studies presented at an NCI-sponsored meeting on July 7, 1998. The data should not be considered final until published in peer-reviewed journals.

Mayo Clinic (Wagner et al., 1999)

Cases were selected from local Minnesota residents who participated in cancer treatment trials at the Mayo Clinic from 1988 through 1994. From a pool of 176 candidates, it was possible to match 61 to similar nontrial patients, with 5 years of follow-up. Cost data were obtained from the Mayo Clinic Multi-Year Population-Based Data Warehouse of Standardized Medical Costs.

Costs for trial patients were modestly higher (3.5%–13% after adjustment for censoring) over follow-up periods ranging from 1 to 5 years. Most of the additional cost for trial participants was incurred during the first few months after enrollment, and the observed cost differences decreased over time.

Group Health Cooperative of Puget Sound (GHC) (Barlow et al., 1998)

Patients in this study were members of GHC who enrolled in Southwest Oncology Group (one of the NCI Cooperative Groups) trials for breast and colorectal cancers from 1990 to 1996. Twenty trial participants with colorectal cancer and 49 with breast cancer were matched to nontrial patients of similar age, time of diagnosis, and initial stage of disease, using an automated matching procedure. Twenty-six of the trial participants with breast cancer were further matched to nontrial patients by medical record review (on co-morbidity and trial eligibility criteria).

Cost data came from the GHC automated cost accounting system. Cumulative costs at 2 years of follow-up were essentially identical for trial and nontrial patients matched by computer. For the 26 pairs of breast cancer patients using closer matching, the mean cost was about $25,000 for nontrial patients and $30,000 for trial patients at 2 years from diagnosis (significant at $p = .04$).

Kaiser Permanente of Northern California (KPNC) (Fireman et al., 1998)

Patients were members of KPNC and participated in any of 10 breast and colorectal cancer trials from 1994 to 1996; 135 were matched to similar nontrial patients. Cost data came from the KPNC automated cost accounting system. The 1-year mean cost was 10 percent higher (about $1,500) for patients in trials. When the 11 patients enrolled in bone marrow transplant trials were excluded from the analysis, the 1-year mean cost for trial patients fell and was slightly lower than, but not statistically significantly different from, costs of patients receiving standard care.

Conclusions

Taken together, these three pilot studies indicate that there may be a modest excess in medical costs for patients enrolled in NCI-sponsored clinical trials, compared with similar patients not enrolled in trials. While these analyses constitute the best data currently available on this question, they were based on small numbers of patients in a few types of cancer treatment trials. A notable finding across the studies was the great variability in treatment costs for patients with the same diagnosis. For these and other reasons, generalizations to other treatment settings, populations, and diseases are not warranted. It remains to be seen whether costs for trial patients are higher, lower, or the same as those for patients outside of a trial, and whether the cost implications can be generalized to other trials.

CLINICAL TRIALS REGISTRY

There is no comprehensive listing of clinical trials in the United States. NIH maintained a clinical trials registry from 1974 to 1979, but now there are only separate NIH registries for trials involving cancer, AIDS, eye conditions, and rare diseases. There are also some small non-NIH registries. As a result, most clinical trials are not listed in any publicly accessible format. This situation is changing, however. There have been calls for a national clinical trials registry from both members of the public and health care providers who want to find out about trials for purposes of enrollment. Further pressure has come from researchers who review evidence from trials and need to know the trials that are ongoing, as well as those that have been completed. These forces led to legislation mandating a U.S. clinical trials registry for serious and life-threatening diseases. The mandate, which appears in Section 113 of the Food and Drug Administration Modernization Act of 1997, calls for the creation of a registry of clinical trials for drugs being carried out under Investigational New Drug (IND) Exemptions. With an additional legislative mandate and funding, this law could become the core of a comprehensive national registry of clinical trials.

A national clinical trials registry is of particular interest to the committee because it would enhance the Health Care Financing Administration's (HCFA's) ability to track the effect of a change in reimbursement policy for clinical trials, as well as audit records to evaluate compliance with the reimbursement rules. The following sections describe the status of the registry as it is developing currently, and the ways in which it should be expanded to serve both as a tool for Medicare and for broader purposes.

Registry of Clinical Trials of Drugs for Serious and Life-Threatening Diseases

The Food and Drug Administration Modernization Act of 1997 (P.L. 105-115) provided for the establishment of an "Information Program on Clinical Trials for Serious or Life-Threatening Diseases" (Section 113). The heart of the program (referred to as a "data bank") is a registry designed to make information about clinical trials of interventions in these diseases widely and easily available to all interested parties: individuals with serious or life-threatening conditions, physicians, researchers, and others. Both publicly funded and industry-funded trials are covered by the mandate, but there is a provision for sponsors to petition for a trial not to be included if they can provide evidence that registration would substantially hinder enrolling participants in the trial. The registry is being developed and will be maintained by the National Library of Medicine (NLM), under the general guidance of the Director of NIH.

A decision about whether to include trials of devices in the registry has been deferred until a report, detailing the potential public health benefits and possible adverse impacts of including device trials, is submitted by DHHS to the Senate Committee on Labor and Human Resources and the House Committee on Commerce. The report is due later in 1999 (two years after passage of the legislation).

Current Status

The registry has so far been carried out as an internal NIH activity, with no formal input from outside NIH. NLM is now establishing the registry, focusing first on NIH-sponsored trials, which are scheduled for complete registration by the end of 1999. They will then take up industry-sponsored trials, as well as the remaining trials funded by public sources (e.g., VA, DoD, CDC), which NLM hopes to enter by the end of the year 2000 (McCray, 1999). However, procedures for identifying and registering industry-sponsored trials have not yet been developed.

Each trial will be assigned a unique identifier. The record will contain the date the trial enters the registry and dates of subsequent modifications (e.g., if eligibility criteria change, or a drug dosage is changed, these changes would have to be reported to the registry), as well as core information items. The legislative mandate requires four pieces of information about each trial:

- description of the purpose of each experimental drug,
- eligibility criteria for participation in the clinical trials,
- location of trial sites, and
- point of contact for those wanting to enroll in the trial.

An NIH working group has developed a somewhat longer (though still brief) list of data elements, but the list is not yet final. Some data items will be required and others optional.

2

Paying for Patient Care in Clinical Trials

The lion's share of funding to carry out clinical trials comes from two main sources: the federal government and private industry. In general, trial budgets cover the costs of setting up and managing the trial, recruiting participants, and collecting and analyzing data. Some money is included to cover special tests and procedures, but this varies. There is an expectation in most cases—more prominent for government-sponsored trials—that at least some, and in many cases most, costs of "routine patient care" will be paid for through the usual mechanism, health insurance.

The Health Care Financing Administration (HCFA) has maintained that some patient care in clinical trials is not reimbursable under Medicare. But HCFA has not issued an explicit policy setting out exactly what should and should not be reimbursed, which has led to varying interpretations of HCFA's intent by its fiscal intermediaries and carriers who process claims, as well as by providers submitting claims.

A large proportion of patient care provided in clinical trials is routine—care that would be eligible for reimbursement if delivered outside of a trial. Although the evidence is limited, it appears that claims for much of this care are submitted to HCFA (and other insurers, for non-Medicare patients) without specifying that the patient is in a clinical trial, and they are paid in the normal course of business by HCFA's contractors.

There is, however, one type of trial for which HCFA has issued explicit guidance: routine care in trials involving certain investigational medical devices became eligible for reimbursement under Medicare in 1995. Other public and private third-party payers have also entered into explicit agreements with the National Institutes of Health (NIH) to provide payment for patient care in selected clinical trials. In some cases payment is limited to routine care, and in others it includes paying for the investigational intervention itself.

Clearly, official policy and common practice and understanding do not always match in reimbursement for patient care costs in clinical trials. In this chapter, we have pieced together as complete a picture as possible of how, and the extent to which, the costs of treating people in clinical trials are actually covered.

CURRENT MEDICARE REIMBURSEMENT RULES RELATING TO INVESTIGATIONAL MEDICAL SERVICES AND CLINICAL TRIALS

The legislation establishing the Medicare program states:

> Notwithstanding any other provisions of this title, no payment may be made for items or services which are not reasonable and necessary for the diagnosis and treatment of illness or injury or to improve the functioning of a malformed body member.

Since the inception of the Medicare program in the mid-1960s, the phrase "reasonable and necessary" has guided Medicare reimbursement. Although little explicit policy has ever been issued on the topic, this clause has been the basis for excluding reimbursement for services in clinical trials. This Medicare interpretation has historical roots in the private insurance sector, whose policies in the 1960s and still, in 1999, exclude coverage of services in clinical trials (GAO, 1999). Most private insurance plans have excluded coverage of services in clinical trials on the basis that the treatment is "experimental" or "investigational," although the language does not explicitly mention clinical trials (GAO, 1999).* However, Medical Directors report that they often approve payment for care in clinical trials on a case-by-case basis. In addition, private insurers have been involved in supporting specific trials (e.g., the Blue Cross/Blue Shield Associa-

---

*The language regarding experimental and investigational treatment in most health insurance contracts is similar to the following, which is taken from a current Group Service Agreement of CIGNA Healthcare of New York, Inc.: "By way of example, but not limitation, the following are specifically excluded services and benefits: "Medical, surgical or other health care procedures and treatments which are experimental or investigational, as determined by the HEALTHPLAN Medical Director in accordance with consensus derived from peer review medical and scientific literature and the practice of the national medical community, including (1) any procedures or treatments which are not recognized as conforming to accepted medical practice; (2) any procedures or treatments in which the scientific assessment of the technique, or its application for a particular condition, has not been completed or its effectiveness has not been established; and (3) any procedures or treatments for which the required approval of a government agency has not been granted at the time the services are rendered." GAO (1999) confirmed in interviews with health plan Medical Directors that this language is interpreted to exclude routine care in clinical trials.

tion was instrumental in initiating a trial of high-dose chemotherapy with bone marrow transplant rescue for women with advanced breast cancer).

Despite the lack of an explicit policy excluding reimbursement for routine care in clinical trials, HCFA has provided clear signals of its intent with regard to reimbursement in events of recent years. First are the events surrounding the 1995 change in policy for reimbursement of services to Medicare beneficiaries in some medical device trials. In 1993, HCFA asked the Office of the Inspector General (OIG) of the Department of Health and Human Services (DHHS) to investigate whether hospitals were billing Medicare "improperly for millions of dollars worth of surgical procedures involving unapproved medical devices," specifically, investigational pacemakers, defibrillators, and other cardiac devices in clinical trials. In a 1996 hearing of the Subcommittee on Investigations of the Senate Committee on Governmental Affairs, an official of the OIG reported their finding that most of the 130 hospitals they investigated had, in fact, improperly billed Medicare for implanting investigational devices. The Inspector General urged HCFA to recover these "overpayments" from the hospitals (Hartwig, 1996).

What might not be clear from the OIG account is that it was not only payment for the investigational devices themselves, but for the implantation procedures, as illustrated by comments of others, including at least one HCFA official.*

---

*This point was made clearly by a HCFA official testifying at the same hearing (Ault, 1996), who stated:

> Medicare's program instructions on medical devices, which were governing until November 1, 1995, were added to the Medicare Hospital Manual, the Carrier Manual, and the Intermediary Manual in 1986. These instructions stated clearly that "medical devices which have not been approved for marketing by the FDA are considered investigational by Medicare and are not reasonable and necessary." The instructions went on to explain that payment would not be made either for the devices or the procedures and services performed using the devices. Additional instructions in these manuals dealing more generally with all noncovered services also state that any services related to a noncovered service are excluded from coverage.
>
> I would like to emphasize that HCFA was clear from the start about its policy regarding both coverage of investigational devices as well as any related services. To provide an example of how the policy was designed to work—if a hospital admission was solely for the purpose of implanting an investigational device, no payment would be made for the hospital stay. On the other hand, if a patient was admitted for chest pain, but it was decided during the visit to implant an investigational device, Medicare would pay for a medical admission recognizing the chest pain, but Medicare would not pay the much higher rate applicable to a surgical stay. No payment would be made for services associated with the surgical procedure to implant the investigational device.

The official also made clear in his testimony that Medicare would have paid for patients in the trials to have the standard device implanted. He said, "We believe that in almost every instance in which an investigational device was provided, hospitals instead could have furnished an approved device, legally billed Medicare for it, and received

By the time of the hearing, HCFA had already changed its policy to allow reimbursement for patients in certain trials involving investigational devices (see below), but not for trials of other types of interventions. The clearest indication that routine patient care still is not considered reimbursable in trials other than those involving devices is found in a 1997 report by the General Accounting Office (GAO, 1997) on reimbursement by HCFA for Medicare beneficiaries in cancer clinical trials. GAO found that reimbursement was, indeed, occurring without HCFA's knowledge (the specific findings are presented later in this chapter). In responding to GAO's draft report, HCFA reported that their actuaries had "nearly doubled their estimates of the extent to which Medicare mistakenly reimburses claims for routine patient care costs. Under HCFA's current policy, any reimbursement for care associated with a cancer clinical trial would be made in error" (GAO, 1997).[*]

HCFA has not issued any new language to change clinical trial reimbursement policy since the 1995 change for trials of medical devices, and no HCFA statements contradictory to what is presented here were found in the course of this study.

Exceptions: Paying Patient Care Costs in Clinical Trials Under Medicare

HCFA can and does make explicit exceptions to its general prohibition against paying for patient care costs in clinical trials. The most far-reaching exception is payment for routine care in a large number of medical device trials conducted under FDA-approved Investigational Device Exemption (IDE) protocols. In addition to medical devices, HCFA has reimbursed for other investigational treatments in specific instances referred to as "coverage with conditions."

Reimbursement for Participants in Clinical Trials Involving Devices Under Medicare

Until 1995, HCFA considered patient care in all trials of unapproved devices to be ineligible for reimbursement under Medicare, as described earlier. This ineligibility extended to trials of approved devices being tested for new uses, even though the same "off label" use would have been reimbursed for patients not in trials. The OIG investigation and its threat of severe economic penalties led hospitals to cease (or at least consider ceasing) participation in device trials. The manufacturers claimed that they were financially incapable of sup-

---

payment. The choice they made, however, was to bill improperly for devices that were part of a clinical trial and therefore not covered."

[*]HCFA's initial estimate was that 25% of Part B claims and 10% of Part A claims for clinical trials were being reimbursed; the revised estimates were 50% and 15%, respectively.

porting the routine patient care costs associated with these trials. The result was an attempt to determine whether it was feasible to extend Medicare coverage to at least some investigational devices while maintaining safe medical care.

In 1995, HCFA's and FDA's interagency agreement changed the reimbursement picture. Device trials under IDEs are now divided into two categories by FDA. Category A involves "experimental," first-of-a-kind devices for which the underlying risk of the device type has not been established for any use. Category B (see Table 2-1) involves "investigational" but not "experimental" devices. These are refinements of approved devices or replications of approved devices by a different manufacturer. Thus, the underlying questions of safety and effectiveness have been answered. A trial is therefore carried out to determine any *incremental risks* or benefits of the new device, or in some cases, simply to obtain approval for marketing. Category A trials continue to be excluded from reimbursement, but category B trials may be eligible for reimbursement. Of the 1,600 IDE trials ongoing (with 250 new ones each year), 96 percent have been placed in category B and 4 percent in category A.

The manufacturers sponsoring trials and the institutions participating in them are responsible for filing paperwork with HCFA and the appropriate Medicare carriers before patients are enrolled. Reimbursement claims for patients who subsequently enter trials are identified by the IDE number assigned by FDA.

Although all category B devices may be eligible for reimbursement, it is not necessarily granted. Decisions not to reimburse for a device can be made at two levels: at HCFA Central Office and at the carrier or fiscal intermediary level. First, HCFA retains the right to declare a specific trial ineligible for coverage, in which case it may issue a policy directive to its carriers and intermediaries informing them of the exclusion. A recent instance involved transmyocardial revascularization using a laser that is approved for other indications. In this case, the evidence for effectiveness was lacking.

Medicare carriers and fiscal intermediaries may exercise their authority to decline reimbursement for particular patients on the basis of "medical necessity." They do not have the authority to countermand a decision by the HCFA Central Office, but they can determine that a particular patient is not eligible for the treatment under Medicare rules. According to a sample of carrier and fiscal intermediary Medical Directors interviewed for this report, they exercise this authority to greater and lesser degrees, with some never refusing reimbursement and others doing so occasionally.

It appears that, overall, the 1995 change in reimbursement rules for devices under IDEs has had the intended effect: treatment of nearly all Medicare patients in eligible trials involving category B devices is reimbursed in a satisfactory manner.

TABLE 2-1. Criteria for Categorization of Investigational Devices[a] Under HCFA/FDA Interagency Agreement

Category A: Experimental	
Subcategory	
1	Class III devices[b] of a type for which no marketing application has been approved for any indication or use
2	Class III devices that would otherwise be in category B but have undergone significant modification for a new indication or use
Category B: Nonexperimental/Investigational	
Subcategory	
1	Devices, regardless of classification, under investigation to establish substantial equivalence to a predicate device (one that is or could be legally marketed)
2	Class III devices whose technological characteristics and indications are comparable to an approved device
3	Class III devices with technological ("generational") advances compared to an approved device
4	Class III devices comparable to an approved device (no significant modifications) but under investigation for a new indication
5	Class III devices on the market before the current regulatory requirements (1976) but now under investigation
6	Devices not posing significant risks (Class I or II) for which an IDE is required

[a]"Note: Some investigational devices may exhibit unique characteristics or raise safety concerns that make additional consideration necessary. For these devices, HCFA and FDA will agree on the additional criteria to be used. FDA will then use these criteria to assign the device to a category. As experience is gained in the categorization process, this attachment may be modified."

[b]Devices are classified by their inherent risks and benefits based on the level of control necessary to assure safety and effectiveness. Class I devices present minimal potential for harm to the user and are subject to only "general controls" (e.g., proper registration and labeling and good manufacturing practices). Class II are those for which general controls alone are insufficient to assure safety and effectiveness, so they are also subject to special controls, which may include special labeling requirements, guidance documents, mandatory performance standards, and postmarket surveillance. Class III is the most stringent regulatory category, including devices for which safety and effectiveness cannot be ensured solely through general or special controls. Class III devices usually support or sustain human life, are of substantial importance in preventing impairment of human health, or present a potential, unreasonable risk of illness or injury. They require premarket approval, which may include evidence from clinical trials.

SOURCE: HCFA/FDA, 1995.

Coverage with Conditions

In certain cases, HCFA has concluded that investigational treatments do meet the test of being "reasonable and necessary" when provided according to certain specifications. An early example of this, starting in 1986, is coverage of the costs of heart transplants only in specific "centers of excellence" according to an approved protocol, and only for patients meeting specified criteria (Evans, 1992). The most prominent current example is a randomized trial of lung volume reduction surgery (LVRS), a relatively new procedure intended to improve lung function and relieve debilitating symptoms for emphysema patients.

By 1995, LVRS was diffusing rapidly—and claims for reimbursement were being submitted to Medicare—despite the lack of evidence from clinical trials that it was an effective treatment. Unanswered questions remained about risk, appropriate selection of patients for surgery, differences in surgical techniques, and qualifications of physicians performing the surgery.

In a 1996 report to HCFA, the Agency for Health Care Policy and Research (AHCPR) concluded that there was insufficient evidence to determine the effectiveness of LVRS (Holohan and Handelsman, 1996). They recommended that HCFA help answer the question of effectiveness by funding the patient care costs for Medicare participants enrolled in a randomized trial of the procedure. HCFA went to the National Heart, Lung and Blood Institute (NHLBI) to develop a study protocol and fund the research portion of what is now the multicenter National Emphysema Treatment Trial. In addition, AHCPR is funding a study of the cost-effectiveness of LVRS as a component of the trial. In this case, no reimbursement is allowed for LVRS for Medicare beneficiaries outside the trial. A determination about effectiveness and appropriate indications (and therefore, Medicare coverage) will be made when the trial is completed (DeParle, 1998).

Simultaneous pancreas-kidney transplants for certain patients with diabetes and end-stage renal disease is another surgical procedure for which insufficient evidence is available to make a general decision about its risks and benefits. Based on an AHCPR recommendation, HCFA is collaborating with the National Institute on Diabetes, Digestive and Kidney Diseases (NIDDK) to provide reimbursement for patients with certain indications who receive their transplants at specific high-volume institutions (in this case, performing at least 30 such procedures per year). The participating transplant centers must also provide data on patients to the NIDDK-supported International Pancreas and Islet Transplant Registry (DeParle, 1998).

Authority of ProPAC to Fund Clinical Trials

Congress at one time recognized the Medicare Program's legitimate interest in collecting information on the safety and effectiveness of new and existing medical services to aid in deciding about whether coverage is warranted. In 1983 amendments to the Medicare section of the Social Security Act, Congress created the independent Prospective Payment Assessment Commission (Pro-PAC) to advise HCFA about hospital payment under Medicare, but also to "identify medically appropriate patterns of health resources use" (42US Code, Sec. 1395ww(e)(6)(E)). ProPAC was also given authority to "carry out, or award grants or contracts for, original research and experimentation, including clinical research, where existing information is inadequate for the development of useful and valid guidelines by the Commission. . . ."

ProPAC never funded any clinical trials. Furthermore, in the Balanced Budget Act of 1997, ProPAC and the Physician Payment Review Commission (which advised on physician payment issues) were merged into the Medicare Payment Advisory Commission and language allowing ProPAC to fund research was eliminated.

THE STATUS QUO IN REIMBURSEMENT

There is relatively little information about how the costs of patient care in clinical trials are actually paid, and the extent to which insurers are paying these costs, either knowingly or unknowingly. What information is available suggests that a sizable proportion is paid for by insurers, including HCFA. This conclusion derives from:

• direct evidence from one study demonstrating that HCFA has paid unknowingly for most routine care of Medicare beneficiaries in certain cancer trials (GAO, 1997),

• evidence that, in the past (before the 1995 change in policy) HCFA unknowingly paid millions of dollars in reimbursement for Medicare beneficiaries in medical device trials (Hartwig, 1996),

• interviews with clinical trial investigators conducted for this study, in which they uniformly acknowledged submitting claims for reimbursement to HCFA and other insurers for routine patient care in trials and getting them paid,

• interviews with private-sector clinical trial sponsors conducted for this study who stated that, while they do cover the costs of "protocol-induced" services, in general they do not provide money to pay for routine patient care; they expect providers to bill insurers for those costs,

• deduction, given the lack of another obvious source of payment for most routine care in trials, and

• lack of evidence from any source that HCFA and other insurers are not reimbursing for this care.

The evidence about payments by HCFA in pre-1995 medical device trials was presented earlier in this chapter. The other points are discussed in the sections that follow. Even though the committee has concluded that a great deal, possibly most, of patient care costs are already reimbursed by Medicare, it acknowledges that not *all* costs are reimbursed. Very little evidence is available about how costs for claims that are denied (or never filed) are eventually paid. Some appear to be absorbed by providers and institutions involved with clinical trials, but at least in some cases, the participant may be left to pay the bill. The committee was presented with anecdotal evidence that participants are sometimes forced unexpectedly to pay large sums for care in clinical trials, although no systematically collected evidence on this could be found. In all that follows, what is missing is any reference to financial burdens on participants.

The GAO Study: Medicare Reimbursement Denials in Cancer Clinical Trials

In February 1997, Senators Mack and Rockefeller first introduced the "Medicare Cancer Clinical Trial Coverage Act" (S. 381), which would have established a demonstration project requiring HCFA to cover routine patient care costs for Medicare beneficiaries enrolled in trials sponsored by the National Cancer Institute (NCI). In order to gauge the potential impact of the legislation (which ultimately did not become law), the Senators asked the General Accounting Office (GAO) to estimate how often claims were denied by HCFA because the costs of treatment were incurred in clinical trials.

The GAO selected a group of cancer trials from NCI's Physician Data Query (PDQ) database that were likely to include people over 65 (GAO, 1997). They focused on trials enrolling patients with cancer of the breast, colon, rectum, prostate, or lung, and limited these to phase 2 and 3 trials, which enroll more patients than do phase 1 trials. All physicians participating in these trials were contacted, and 186 (55 percent) of them responded. These physicians had enrolled 1,143 patients into the trials between March 1 and September 30, 1996, including 217 Medicare beneficiaries. (One physician reported automatically excluding Medicare beneficiaries from clinical trials because of concerns over reimbursement.) The Medicare carrier paid the claims in all but eight cases. Those eight had been treated by the same physician and, for seven of them, the claims denied were for chemotherapy and other drugs.

In this study, when providers submitted claims for patients in cancer clinical trials (as long as that fact was not acknowledged), they were rarely denied. This is one small study, but it is the only one of its kind.

How Clinical Trial Providers Recoup Patient Care Costs

There are no published studies on how the costs of caring for patients in clinical trials are covered, although there is a widespread understanding that third-party payers do, indeed, pay for much of this care. The committee commissioned a small study to gather information on this question (Dobson and Sturm, 1999). The Lewin Group interviewed 12 individuals with experience organizing and conducting clinical trials, asking generally about how they sought reimbursement for enrolled patients. (They did not request or receive billing or accounts data for specific trials.) In addition, the Lewin Group report summarized a survey of 17 oncology practices conducted for the American Society of Clinical Oncology (ASCO) concerning how they would seek reimbursement for patients treated in a hypothetical clinical trial protocol.

The results of the interviews should be treated as glimpses into the subject of reimbursement for patients in clinical trials, not a comprehensive—or even representative—set of data. The individuals interviewed spoke only for themselves. The committee makes no claims of generalizability, but it is worth noting that the interviewees were speaking from direct, current experience. The results of both the interviews and the survey are presented without identifying the respondents.

Those interviewed by the Lewin Group were:

• representatives of large pharmaceutical and medical device companies with experience sponsoring numerous clinical trials for the Medicare population;
• the director of a private research institute that serves as a site for several multisite clinical trials;
• the director of clinical research and the national director of clinical resources at a federal agency that sponsors clinical trials;
• the manager of cardiology trials at a major academic medical center (AMC);
• the director of a large clinical research center at a major AMC;
• the administrative manager of a general clinical research center (GCRC) at a major AMC;
• the director of a clinical research committee at a major AMC, who is also a former member of an Institutional Review Board.

Findings from the interviews and the ASCO survey are reported from the perspectives of oncology, cardiology, NIH GCRCs, and the medical device and pharmaceutical industries.

Oncology

Oncologists commonly bill third-party payers for both investigational and routine patient care costs in clinical trials. One interviewee believes this is, at least in part, because the definition of what is "investigational" and what is "routine" is not clear for many types of cancer that generally defy treatment.

For example, no standard treatment exists for advanced melanoma, so it is difficult to decide which services and tests are standard or routine treatment and which are investigational or research-related. Even though no standard currently exists, patients not enrolled in a clinical trial are still seen and treated by physicians prescribing their own idiosyncratic "routine" care that would be billed to third-party payers. In a sense, all treatments for these patients are investigational, whether or not formally labeled as clinical research. Thus, in advanced melanoma trials, because no standard exists, oncologists generally classify some patient care costs as "routine" and seek reimbursement from insurers.

Oncologists also sometimes submit claims to Medicare and other insurers for tests (e.g., liver function tests and computed tomography [CT] scans) done more frequently in clinical trials than they might otherwise be performed. They may also bill for components of complex treatments, such as bone marrow transplantation for unproven indications, without specifying the procedure itself.

The ASCO survey presented 17 clinical oncology practices (12 group practices, 2 academic medical centers, and 2 managed care organizations) with a mock protocol for a phase 3 trial of a chemotherapy drug for prostate cancer. The mock protocol was designed to resemble a "typical" oncology trial and gave a detailed account of the trial background, the eligibility and exclusion criteria, and the schedule of required studies and tests. The tests and services included in this survey ranged from office visits and clinical labs to chest X-rays and CT scans. The oncology practices were then asked for which services/tests in this clinical trial they would "normally bill" an insurer, assuming first industry sponsorship and then NIH sponsorship.

The responses indicate that oncologists in academic medical centers and group practices would bill for patient care services in both industry- and NIH-sponsored clinical trials for substantial portions of patient care costs. Claims would be submitted for nearly all office visits and clinical laboratory services, and for 50 to 70 percent of chest X-rays, CT scans, and bone scans.

Cardiology

Cardiologists commonly bill insurers for routine patient care costs in clinical trials. In at least some sites, however, costs for procedures mandated by the protocol but not necessarily required for standard patient treatment ("protocol-induced costs") are not submitted for reimbursement and are usually covered by research dollars.

In clinical trials comparing two standard treatments for coronary artery disease, such as percutaneous transluminal coronary angioplasty (PTCA) and pharmacological therapies, both treatments would be reimbursable by most third-party payers outside the scope of a trial. Therefore, routine patient care associated with both treatments is billed as though there were no clinical trial.

The investigators interviewed stated that to cover trial costs, physicians seek insurer reimbursement for some patient care costs, and also cross-subsidize from other sources of revenue. In this case, other sources of revenue might include enrolling in better-funded industry-sponsored trials or affiliating with organizations that bring in money from clinical care.

General Clinical Research Centers

GCRCs are NIH-funded hospital beds set aside specifically for research, which can be used by investigators supported by the NIH, as well as those funded by other public and private agencies. Most GCRC studies are early (phase 1) studies, with intensive medical treatment, monitoring, or both. GCRCs use rigorous guidelines and procedures to sort out the costs of "routine" versus "experimental" patient care. For example, in one GCRC at a major academic medical center, all GCRC patient bills are tagged before reimbursement. The tag diverts the patient's bill to the GCRC administrative research office before being forwarded to the insurer. There the staff reviews the patient's category assignment and compares each line charge on the patient's bill to the trial protocol to see which charges are mandated by the protocol and which charges are "non-research" related costs. In this way, the GCRC identifies two types of costs that are not reimbursed by third-party insurers: (1) research costs for unproven therapies or diagnostic techniques, and (2) "usual" or "routine" care costs, which are part of the research project, for patients who would not otherwise have been hospitalized or received such care except for their participation in the research study.

The consensus from other interviews was that GCRCs are not representative of most research sites in that they dedicate a substantial amount of money to the administration of a proper billing system for routine patient care costs in clinical trials. Most research sites interviewed felt that it would be impractical for them to fund the administrative system and staff employed by the GCRCs to ensure proper billing.

Medical Device Industry

Most routine patient care costs for clinical trials of FDA-designated "category B" devices are paid for by all third-party payers, but payment is not guaranteed. An example reported by one interviewee is a category B defibrillator trial in which third-party reimbursement was received for 85 percent of the patients. In the 15 percent of unreimbursed cases, the insurer decided against paying on the basis that the device was not "medically necessary," not that it was experimental. Both Medicare beneficiaries and privately insured patients were in this clinical trial, and overall, Medicare was more likely to provide reimbursement than were the private insurers.

Pharmaceutical Industry

Policies on how patient care costs are paid in industry-sponsored clinical trials differ by company. In general, however, pharmaceutical sponsors give physicians more money per patient than nonindustry sponsors for both data management and clinical care. The ASCO survey found that the median NCI payment is $750 per patient versus $2,500 per patient for industry-sponsored trials. Pharmaceutical sponsors usually cover costs for all procedures, both routine and investigational, required by the protocol. Routine costs not required by the protocol are commonly billed to third-party payers and are paid by the pharmaceutical sponsor only if reimbursement is denied by the insurer (this varies from company to company).

In a real example of an industry-sponsored clinical trial, a drug is tested to treat benign prostate disease and lower urinary tract symptoms. In this case, surgery is the standard treatment the patient would have received outside of the trial. Costs associated with the standard surgery in the comparison arm of the study are billed to a third-party payer, while all experimental costs for patient care and additional procedures required by the protocol are borne by the company.

Treatment of Clinical Trial Claims by Medicare Fiscal Intermediaries and Carriers

To find out how Medicare policy on clinical trials is implemented, the Institute of Medicine (IOM) project staff conducted semistructured telephone interviews with several Medical Directors of Medicare fiscal intermediaries and carriers around the country. HCFA, in its Medicare manuals, regulations, and other types of specific written guidance, sets the rules for reimbursement of medical services for Medicare beneficiaries. But the day-to-day decisions about reimbursement for hospital and physician services are made by Medicare fiscal intermediaries and carriers, acting as agents for Medicare Parts A and B, respectively. Because HCFA does not issue specific guidance on each and every service, these insurers have a certain amount of discretion to determine what will and will not be paid for, based on their understanding of the Medicare rules.

In the case of clinical trials, fiscal intermediary and carrier Medical Directors in different parts of the country share a general understanding that at least some services—including possibly some entire episodes of care—are excluded from Medicare reimbursement because they do not meet the "reasonable and necessary" criteria. However, the Medical Directors vary in their interpretation of what they would and would not consider covered in the context of clinical trials. The information reported here derives from discussions of hypothetical claims situations and not an analysis of actual reimbursement decisions.

In conversations with Medical Directors, there was a general recognition that providers submit claims for beneficiaries in clinical trials, most of which do not specify (through coding conventions) that the individual was in a trial. The Medical Directors all believed such claims to be relatively few.

Occasionally, claims are submitted that raise the possibility that the patient is in an investigational protocol; for example, if an administered drug is unnamed or designated as unapproved; if the claim is for the administration of chemotherapy, but there is no drug charge; or if a medication is paired with an unusual diagnosis. These cases might be investigated and the fact of a clinical trial uncovered.

No Medical Directors said they would flatly deny reimbursement for any and all patients in clinical trials, but their thresholds between reimbursement and no reimbursement varied. Several hypothetical scenarios were discussed, eliciting a range of responses, summarized in the next section. It should be noted that these are responses that would be made if the Medical Director was aware that treatment had been given in the context of a trial, which, according to those interviewed, would be the exception rather than the rule.

All Clinical Trials Except Those Involving Devices

Randomized clinical trial comparing two or more standard treatments. There was total agreement that it was appropriate to reimburse for routine care of all Medicare patients enrolled. Source of trial sponsorship would not affect the decision.

Randomized clinical trial comparing standard treatment with an investigational treatment. Most would reimburse for routine care of patients receiving standard treatment but not the investigational arm (some, however, would provide some reimbursement for standard elements of the investigational treatment). One Medical Director would decline payment for all aspects of both the investigational and control arm of such a trial.

Phase 1 and 2 cancer clinical trials. Responses ranged from blanket denial of all claims to full reimbursement if drugs were approved and accepted off-label for the indication. Acceptance for off-label use would be based on listing in standard compendia. If a trial involved both approved and unapproved drugs, some would reimburse for treatment with approved drugs but not unapproved ones, and others would reimburse nothing for the treatment episode.

Clinical Trials Involving Devices

Medical Directors shared the understanding that devices classified by FDA as "category A" were not eligible for reimbursement, but that those in "category B" were eligible, subject to carriers' discretion. Instances were also cited in which HCFA had issued directives that procedures involving certain category B devices not be reimbursed (e.g., laser transmyocardial revascularization), and these directives were routinely followed by carriers. The Medical Directors were asked whether they distinguished among the subclasses of category B devices, but otherwise were not presented with scenarios. As with non-device trials, there was some variation in how Medicare reimbursement requirements were interpreted.

The Medical Directors believe they are generally more aware of patients treated under IDEs than in other types of clinical trials because of the specific payment rules for device trials. In practice, some virtually never deny a reimbursement claim for a category B device (except in the case of explicit HCFA guidance against reimbursement). At the other extreme, one Medical Director reported denying 10–20 such claims per month. Those denials are based on a determination that the device was not "medically necessary" for those patients.

General Observations

The rules about reimbursement for treatment in clinical trials under Medicare are open to interpretation, but to no greater degree than other reimbursement situations, according to the Medical Directors interviewed. They stressed that HCFA does not provide specific, detailed guidance for each hypothetical situation. The vast majority of claims are routine, however, and require no special attention. Claims involving clinical trials are a tiny fraction of the claims flowing through these offices, and even among claims requiring individual decisions, they do not appear to be a major problem for Medical Directors.

According to those interviewed, although fiscal intermediaries and carriers retain substantial discretion over reimbursement decisions, these decisions have become more uniform over time, for several reasons. One reason is that the number of fiscal intermediaries and carriers has been steadily reduced since the inception of Medicare, with larger and larger areas covered by each one. In addition, there is increased consultation and collaboration among these entities, and reimbursement criteria and decisions are a frequent source of discussion.

Medical Directors also noted the inconsistency that sometimes occurs when reimbursement is provided for use of an inpatient drug for an off-label indication outside of a clinical trial, while the same claim would be denied if the treatment were given in a clinical trial. The same might be true of new or modified procedures that might not be fully detailed in a routine claim but would be obvious and not reimbursable if part of a clinical trial.

PROGRAMS AND PROPOSALS FOR REIMBURSING
PATIENT CARE COSTS IN CLINICAL TRIALS

Since the mid-1990s, various agreements have been struck and legislation introduced to pay for some patient care costs in some clinical trials. Each of the arrangements included here was considered by the committee in its deliberations, although the reimbursement recommendations proposed in this report differ in significant ways from those described.

DoD/NCI Agreement

In January 1996, the Department of Defense (DoD) began a 3-year demonstration project to pay medical costs for cancer patients who enrolled in phase 2 or 3 NCI-sponsored cancer treatment trials (DoD/NCI, 1996). All services associated with treatment in the trial are paid for, including:

- diagnostic testing and evaluation required to determine whether a patient meets the eligibility criteria,
- chemotherapeutic agents, except investigational agents,
- treatment of complications, and
- follow-up and testing after active treatment period.

As of April 1999, 206 patients had participated in this program during its first 2 ½ years (out of about 11,760 TRICARE-eligible patients diagnosed with cancer each year). More than half (113) had breast cancer, and the rest had a variety of other cancers. Roughly two-thirds were in phase 2 trials and one-third in phase 3 trials.

Information about specific treatments was not available for the entire participating group, but during the initial year and a half of the program, when the first 125 were treated, 91 patients had entered trials that included bone marrow transplantation (73 for solid tumors and 18 for hematologic malignancies).

It appears that the DoD benefit was seen as a means to enter trials with treatment including bone marrow transplantation, which, for the solid tumors, would have been some form of high-dose therapy with autologous bone marrow rescue. Most patients were in phase 2 trials, so entry would not have required randomization, which might have meant accepting standard treatment without a bone marrow transplant. No economic analyses were completed to determine the cost of this program because of the small numbers of participants and the skewed distribution toward bone marrow transplantation (Szymanski, 1999).

The demonstration project with NCI has been extended in time and expanded in 1999 to include coverage of patient care costs in cancer prevention trials (DoD 1999). NCI has requested coverage of phase 1 trials as well, but DoD has decided not to include them at this time. DoD has also considered expanding coverage to NIH-sponsored trials for medical conditions other than cancer but has not yet done so.

VA/NCI Agreement

The Department of Veterans Affairs (VA) and NCI signed a 3-year agreement in January 1997 under which VA agreed to pay for medical care in NCI-sponsored clinical trials for veterans in the VA health care system (VA/NCI, 1997). The agreement provides for payment in trials at VA medical centers and at non-VA sites, but in practice, VA has limited coverage to NCI-sponsored trials at its own facilities (exceptions could still be made, e.g., in the case of a rare tumor for which no trials are ongoing at VA facilities). A direct per-case reimbursement arrangement was set up for VA physicians to encourage increased participation.

VA-eligible individuals may enter trials in cancer prevention, diagnosis, and treatment, including all phases of trials. All services required by the trials are paid for by VA, which is consistent with their provision of all necessary medical care at no cost to beneficiaries.

As of early 1999, VA was not tracking either the number of individuals enrolled through this agreement, or the costs of treatment for patients enrolled in trials.

AAHP/NIH Agreement

The American Association of Health Plans (AAHP) is a trade organization comprising more than 1,000 managed care health plans of all types, with combined coverage of more than 100 million people. In December 1998, AAHP signed an agreement with NIH designed to increase participation of member plan enrollees in NIH-sponsored trials (AAHP, 1998). AAHP will encourage plans to reimburse the costs of routine patient care for people enrolled in trials, up to about the same amount they would reimburse for the costs of standard treatment outside a trial. For trials in which treatment is substantially more expensive than standard care, plans will be encouraged to work with NIH to determine the best sources for covering additional costs. The agreement also includes provisions for monitoring the impact of new reimbursement provisions and for research on the role of clinical trials in health care.

AAHP member plans are all independent and not obligated to change their policy regarding clinical trials. No reports on implementation of the agreement are yet available.

UnitedHealth Group

UnitedHealth Group (UHG), a large managed care provider, began in January 1999 offering reimbursement for participants in certain cancer trials conducted under the auspices of the NCI-sponsored Coalition of National Cancer Cooperative Groups. According to the UHG Medical Director, "UHG grants an exception to the 'investigational' clause for any health plan member who enrolls in one of the Coalition's multicenter trials" (Newcomer, 1999). During the first 8 months of the program, few individuals took advantage of the benefit—fewer than 10 UHG patients entered eligible trials (Newcomer, 1999).

State Laws

Several states have enacted laws that require private insurers (i.e., not HCFA) to reimburse the costs of routine patient care in certain types of clinical trials. Rhode Island has the oldest law, requiring insurers to cover the patient care costs for beneficiaries enrolled in NIH-sponsored cancer clinical trials. Beginning in 1991, patients in phase 3 and 4 trials were eligible. Coverage was extended subsequently to phase 2 trials. The law has no reporting requirements, and the state has not kept track of how many clinical trial participants have been in trials and had their care reimbursed as a result of the law.

In January 1999, a Maryland law went into effect providing reimbursement of costs in all phases of cancer trials, as well as phase 2, 3, and 4 trials for "any other life-threatening condition" sponsored by major government agencies or by industry, under an FDA-approved Investigational New Drug Exemption (IND). Patients must be treated in an institution with a "multiple project assurance contract," which currently limits treatment in the state to the University of Maryland and Johns Hopkins University hospitals.

The Maryland law also requires an annual report on the patients in clinical trials covered during the previous year, to be prepared by the state insurance commissioner based on information provided by the insurers. In addition, the commissioner is required to create a Workgroup on Insurance Coverage for Patient Care Cost in Clinical Trials, which is charged with, at a minimum, developing methodology to assess the economic and clinical impact of coverage under the law.

A Virginia law requiring reimbursement for treatment in cancer clinical trials took effect in July 1999. Eligibility by sponsor and host institution is similar to the Maryland law. A Georgia law went into effect on July 1, 1998 requiring insurers to reimburse routine medical costs for children treated in phase 2 and 3 clinical trials. No information is currently available on the results of any of these state programs.

Selected Proposed National Legislation

Legislation has been proposed in the current and previous Congresses to provide reimbursement for routine patient care costs for Medicare beneficiaries enrolled in cancer clinical trials of varying sponsorship, and for coverage of routine patient care for nonelderly individuals with private insurance enrolled in clinical trials for serious and life-threatening medical conditions.

The major bill aimed at Medicare is called the "Medicare Cancer Clinical Trial Coverage Act" and has been introduced several times, including the current congressional session. This bill proposes covering "routine patient care costs" in cancer trials sponsored by NIH, VA, DoD, industry (for trials under INDs or IDEs), and other NIH-supported private institutions. The bill defines the covered costs to be limited to those covered by Medicare under standard treatment conditions (i.e., outside of clinical trials).

Provisions for some clinical trial coverage by private insurers have been included in all recent versions of the "Patients' Bill of Rights." The bill passed by the House of Representatives in October 1999 would cover routine patient care in government-sponsored trials for "life-threatening or serious illness for which no standard treatment is effective" (H.R. 358). The bill passed by the Senate in July 1999 (S. 240) contains a narrower provision, including only clinical trials for cancer treatment. The bills also require the Secretary of HHS to carry out a formal rulemaking process to develop "standards relating to the coverage of routine patient costs" for clinical trial participants. This would involve appointment of a committee and facilitator who would report on what the standards should be.

$$\wp \quad \wp \quad \wp$$

APPENDIX: A PRIMER ON MEDICARE

Title XVIII of the Social Security Act, entitled "Health Insurance for the Aged and Disabled"—commonly known as Medicare—provides health insurance for people in the United States who:

- are at least 65 years old,
- are disabled, or
- have permanent kidney failure.

When first passed in 1965, Medicare covered only people 65 and older. The other groups became eligible as a result of legislation in 1973. The Medicare program now covers 95 percent of the aged population, plus many persons who are on Social Security because of disability. In 1997, about 38 million enrollees were covered, and benefit payments averaged about $6,300 per enrollee. Total disbursements were $214 billion.

The two main parts of Medicare are "Part A"—Hospital Insurance, which covers most inpatient care—and "Part B"—Supplementary Medical Insurance, which mainly covers physician fees and outpatient care.

Most people pay no premiums for Part A because they have earned the right to coverage through working. Premiums are charged for Part B, amounting to 25 percent of the average expenditure for beneficiaries.

The Benefits

Part A Covered Services

Inpatient hospital care in a semiprivate room, meals, regular nursing services, operating and recovery room, intensive care, inpatient prescription drugs, laboratory tests, X-rays, psychiatric hospital, inpatient rehabilitation, long-term care hospitalization, and other services and supplies are covered. Part A does not cover physician services, which are covered under Part B.

Beneficiaries pay a deductible ($764 in 1998) and nothing more for the first 60 days of inpatient hospital care each year. Starting at 60 days, there is a daily copayment through 90 days, after which Medicare coverage either ends or the beneficiary may use "lifetime reserve days," which require a copayment.

Skilled nursing facility (SNF) care within 30 days (generally) of a hospitalization that lasts at least three days is covered. Covered services are similar to those for inpatient hospital care, but also include rehabilitation and appliances. Up to 100 days are allowed per episode of care, with full coverage for the first 20 days and a daily copayment after that.

Home Health Agency (HHA) care is covered for home-bound beneficiaries who need intermittent or part-time skilled nursing or certain other therapy or rehabilitation care, according to a plan of treatment (and periodic review) prepared by a physician. (The few beneficiaries with no Part A insurance receive HHA coverage under Part B.) Some medical supplies and durable medical equipment are also covered. Full-time nursing care, food, blood, and drugs are not covered services. HHA care has no duration limitations, no copayment, and no deductible. Beneficiaries pay a 20 percent coinsurance for durable medical equipment. (Between 1998 and 2003, a portion of HHA care will be transferred to Part B for payment.)

Hospice care is available to beneficiaries with a life expectancy of six months or less who elect to forgo further potentially curative medical treatment, and receive only hospice care. Such care includes pain relief, supportive medical and social services, physical therapy, nursing services, and symptom management for a terminal illness. There is no deductible for hospice care, but beneficiaries pay a very small coinsurance amount for drugs and for inpatient respite care.

Part B Covered Services

- physician services (in both hospital and nonhospital settings),
- clinical laboratory and diagnostic tests,
- durable medical equipment and most supplies,
- diagnostic tests,
- ambulance services,
- flu vaccinations,
- prescription drugs that cannot be self-administered,
- certain self-administered anticancer drugs, and
- blood not supplied as part of inpatient hospital care.

Beneficiaries pay an annual deductible, monthly premiums, and coinsurance for services (usually 20 percent of the Medicare allowed charges). There is a separate deductible for blood. For end-stage renal disease patients, Medicare covers kidney dialysis and physician charges related to kidney transplants and follow-up care.

Medicare+Choice

Under Medicare+Choice, beneficiaries may opt for a capitated health plan instead of the traditional fee-for-service program. These plans must provide all standard Medicare benefits, but may offer additional benefits.

Services not Covered

Some health care services are not provided as a basic benefit under any part of Medicare (although some or all may be included in managed care plans). These include

- long-term nursing care or custodial care,
- most dental care,
- certain other health care needs (e.g., dentures, eyeglasses, hearing aids),

and

- most prescription drugs.

Organization of Care and Payments to Health Care Providers

Most Medicare beneficiaries get care in the "traditional" fee-for-service environment—they go to doctors and institutions of their choosing, Medicare pays the government's share, and, if required, the beneficiary pays his or her share. Physicians are paid the lesser of either the submitted charges or a fee schedule based on a "relative value scale." Fee schedules also govern payment for durable medical equipment and clinical laboratory services. Historically, various hospital outpatient, SNF, and HHA services have been paid through a somewhat complicated mix of systems, but prospective payment systems are being phased in for these services, as directed by the Balanced Budget Act of 1997.

Under Medicare+Choice, prepaid managed care plans operate much like managed care in the private insurance market. Medicare pays a set amount for each person enrolled, and the plan is responsible for coordinating all services for the beneficiary. With some exceptions, the beneficiary is limited to a certain set of physicians and must abide by certain rules that may restrict choice (e.g., requiring referral from a primary care provider to see a specialist). In order to attract enrollees, most managed care plans offer benefits not covered under fee-for-service Medicare (e.g., coverage of most Medicare cost-sharing, expanded preventive care, prescription drugs, eyeglasses, dental care, or hearing aids). Payments to the Medicare+Choice plans are based on a blend of local and national capitated rates, and vary based on characteristics of the enrolled population.

Medicare Financing

All financial operations for Medicare are handled through two trust funds, one for Part A and one for Part B. The trust funds are maintained as special accounts in the U.S. Treasury and are credited with all income receipts and charged with all Medicare expenditures for benefits and administration costs. Extra funds not needed for the payment of costs are invested in special Treasury Securities.

Most of the money to fund Part A comes from a mandatory payroll deduction for almost all U.S. workers. These contributions pay the expenses of current beneficiaries and serve to qualify those contributing for benefits when they become eligible for Medicare.

Part B is funded by beneficiary premiums, which are set to cover 25 percent of average per capita Medicare expenditures. Nearly all the rest comes from general U.S. Treasury funds (i.e., tax revenues).

Medicare Claims Processing

Medicare claims are processed regionally by private insurance companies under contract to HCFA. "Fiscal intermediaries" process Part A claims, and "carriers" process claims for part B. They apply the Medicare coverage rules to determine the appropriateness of claims and issue payments to providers for the government.

Peer Review Organizations

Each state has a HCFA-funded Peer Review Organization (PRO), consisting of health care practitioners who evaluate the general quality of care provided to Medicare beneficiaries and carry out programs to improve the quality of services. PROs are also a contact point for beneficiaries who have complaints about their care and may run programs to educate beneficiaries about the program and their rights and responsibilities.

Medicare Administration

HCFA, within DHHS, has primary responsibility for Medicare, including formulation of reimbursement and coverage policy and guidelines, but other entities have specific roles to play. The Social Security Administration determines an individual's initial Medicare entitlement and maintains the Medicare master beneficiary record.

A Board of Trustees, with two appointed public members and four ex-officio members, oversees the financial operations of the Medicare trust funds. The Secretary of the Treasury is the managing trustee. The board reports on the status and operation of the Medicare trust funds to Congress each year.

State agencies (usually state Health Departments under agreements with HCFA) help DHHS survey, inspect, and certify health care facilities or institutions that participate in the Medicare program.

SOURCE: Adapted from "Medicare: A Brief Summary," available at www. hcfa.gov/medicare/ormedmed.htm#medicare.

Recommendations for Medicare Clinical Trial Reimbursement

Clinical trials have become an essential component of modern medical care because they are the best means of finding out which health care interventions work and which do not. Trials produce information of value to future patients, and frequently benefit the people enrolled in them. Medicare beneficiaries and taxpayers have a shared interest in the development of reliable information about health care interventions, because such information provides the basis for rational health care and resource allocation decisions by providers and patients.

Although neither regulations nor specific policy directives have been issued about the reimbursement of routine patient care costs in clinical trials, the impression is widespread that the Medicare statute excludes from reimbursement all or some such costs (see chapter 2). This impression is apparent from the nature of legislation introduced in Congress to assure reimbursement for routine patient care costs, from statements of HCFA officials, and from remarks of providers. In chapter 2, the committee also established that, in practice, Medicare reimburses many claims for routine patient care. Thus, a wide gap separates many people's impressions of HCFA's rules and the demonstrable facts of actual reimbursement.

The committee is recommending explicit policy to legitimize reimbursement for much—though not all—of the care rendered to participants in clinical trials. Reimbursement should not be denied solely because the care is delivered as part of a clinical trial. In addition, the recommendations apply to all clinical trials involving any type of intervention in any aspect of health care and for any illness, for care that would be eligible for Medicare reimbursement outside of trials. They apply whether government, industry, or other private sources support or sponsor the trial.

Medicare reimbursement should not hinge on a judgment by HCFA about the quality of the trial. However, HCFA does have a legitimate interest in assuring that trials meet currently accepted standards for scientific merit and protection of research participants. The committee recommends limiting reimbursement to trials that have been reviewed and accepted by all relevant institutional review boards (IRBs). The committee does not believe that HCFA should evaluate every trial for which a reimbursement claim is submitted, but it should have access to documentation of a trial's scientific merit and the fact of IRB approval, upon request. The committee believes the need for such review would be quite rare.

A new reimbursement policy following these recommendations would satisfy two conditions the committee believes to be key: (1) beneficiaries would not be denied reimbursement merely because they have volunteered to participate in a clinical trial; (2) the new rules would not impose excessive administrative burdens on HCFA, its fiscal intermediaries and carriers, or investigators, providers, or participants in clinical trials. Explicit rules would have the added benefit of increasing the uniformity of reimbursement decisions made by Medicare fiscal intermediaries and carriers in different parts of the country. Greater uniformity would, in turn, decrease the uncertainty about reimbursement when providers and patients embark on a clinical trial.

The fundamental principle is that reimbursement decisions should be made independent of whether a beneficiary is receiving care in or out of a clinical trial. Reimbursement should be provided for all services to which the beneficiary would be generally entitled under Medicare. This rule would provide reimbursement for a large share of services to participants in clinical trials.

The fundamental rule would apply to routine care in all trials comparing standard approved interventions (drugs, devices, procedures, or other). It also would apply to routine care in trials of new versus standard drugs. No new reimbursement policy is needed for routine care in trials of most investigational medical devices. Under the 1995 agreement between FDA and HCFA, reimbursement for participants in trials of devices is allowed when the device is "investigational," but not when it is "experimental" (i.e., when the device itself is not a new type but is a modified version of an existing approved device or is being used for a new indication). For such devices the underlying questions of safety and effectiveness have already been answered. Such devices are classified in "category B." Devices for which initial questions of safety and effectiveness have not been answered are designated "category A."

The committee believes that reimbursement should be provided for procedures under rules analogous to those applied to medical devices; procedures that are modifications of, or new uses for existing procedures should be reimbursed at the same level as the existing, accepted procedure. Conversely, as with category A devices, Medicare should not pay routinely for procedures that are considered "experimental," although HCFA may (and should) choose to do so in specific trials. The committee recognizes that classifying procedures may be challenging. A "gray zone" in which a reimbursement decision is unclear will require some special determinations by HCFA. Nonetheless, this provision is an essential component of the overall recommendation.

In addition to providing reimbursement through the proposed policies, the committee urges HCFA to use its existing authority to support selected trials and in two ways to assist in the development of new trials. First, HCFA should reimburse for care in selected trials that would not otherwise qualify, or reimburse at a higher rate than would otherwise be allowed for investigational interventions that are more expensive than the standard treatment. Second, HCFA should assist in the development of new trials of particular importance to the Medicare population.

In all cases, HCFA should provide clear guidance on how the recommended reimbursement policies should be implemented by providers and the entities that process Medicare claims. Such guidance would promote nationally uniform administration and minimize uncertainty for providers and patients about what will and will not be reimbursed.

Finally, although not a requirement of implementing a new policy, the committee recommends prompt completion of a national clinical trials registry. Such a registry will increase HCFA's ability to monitor reimbursement for services in clinical trials, in addition to serving its other functions.

RECOMMENDATIONS

RECOMMENDATION 1. Medicare should reimburse routine care for patients in clinical trials in the same way it reimburses routine care for patients not in clinical trials.

This principle applies to payments for physicians and other providers, routine laboratory and other diagnostic tests, and any other services that comprise routine care for a given patient. All coverage and medical necessity rules and all other restrictions that apply to patients not in clinical trials would apply to care in clinical trials.

The committee recommends a broad definition of clinical trials—including all phases and legitimate designs and all sources of sponsorship (government, industry, or other)—all of which should be equally eligible for reimbursement. This definition does not mean, however, that any treatment simply called a "clinical trial" would qualify for reimbursement. To qualify, a clinical trial must have a written protocol that describes a scientifically sound study and have been approved by all relevant IRBs before participants are enrolled. HCFA should articulate criteria for an acceptable trial and IRB review, which investigators would apply to determine whether their studies are eligible for reimbursement. (HCFA could state the criteria in terms of "current NIH standards," e.g., rather than stating specific study characteristics.) The committee recognizes that controversies surround both the quality of current clinical trials and IRBs, but holds that these issues are being addressed in various ways by DHHS and other sectors of government, and should not be addressed routinely in HCFA's reimbursement decisions.

Medicare should reimburse routine patient care costs, but not all costs in clinical trials. Medicare should not reimburse the costs of experimental interventions (except category B devices for which reimbursement is allowed under agreement with FDA, and certain procedures as described in recommendation 2), of data collection and record keeping that would not be required but for the trial, or of other services to clinical trial participants necessary solely to satisfy data collection needs of the clinical trial ("protocol-induced costs"). These costs should remain the responsibility of research sponsors, private and public.

Medicare should continue its current practice of reimbursing costs of treating conditions that result as unintended consequences (complications) of clinical trials.

RECOMMENDATION 2. HCFA should reimburse surgeons (or other practitioners) for treating patients in randomized clinical trials involving procedures that are variations or modifications of accepted procedures, or new uses for accepted procedures.

Under the current interpretation of Medicare reimbursement rules, the committee believes that surgeons and others performing surgical or other procedures in trials might not be eligible to be reimbursed for those services. Therefore, the committee recommends that procedures that have become widely accepted as a part of standard medical practice, but which, as part of a clinical trial, are being rigorously evaluated, or are being modified or applied for new indications to determine the incremental risks and benefits, should be eligible for reimbursement at the rate for the standard procedure. Conversely, types of procedures for which initial questions of safety and efficacy have not been resolved would not be eligible for reimbursement.

Unlike the basic recommendation regarding routine patient care costs, which applies to all clinical trials, this recommendation would limit reimbursement to randomized trials (the equivalent of "phase 3" trials for drugs and devices). The committee believes this limitation is appropriate in order to avoid providing reimbursement for uncontrolled experimentation by practitioners. The introduction of new drugs and devices is governed by FDA under a formal system that involves phased trials (see chapter 1). In contrast, the introduction of new procedures is not governed by any regulatory authority. In their early phases, procedures are modified or tried for different indications in clinical practice, but rarely in formal trials. However, once a new or modified procedure has been defined and developed to the point that it is distinct enough from the predicate procedure, it may be tested against the standard treatment (the predicate procedure or other accepted treatment) in a formal randomized trial. Medicare should provide reimbursement to the surgeon or other practitioner for treating patients in such trials.

Further clarification may be needed to make clear the committee's intent with regard to reimbursement for procedures on patients in clinical trials. The committee is expressing no judgments about when trials of procedures should or should not be carried out, or who should be involved in them if they are. This recommendation is not intended to influence the criteria or processes HCFA uses to decide on coverage of new procedures under usual medical care. It applies only when a trial of a procedure is being done—for the all the reasons that trials are done—and claims for reimbursement for the procedure are submitted by practitioners.

HCFA's initial task in implementing this recommendation will be to develop definitions for classifying procedures analogous to "category A" and "category B" devices. These definitions describing what is and is not allowed will be applied in the field when claims are submitted. HCFA should not be required to rule routinely on the eligibility of procedures before bills may be submitted. In the same way that providers are responsible for following reimbursement rules for all services under Medicare, they will be responsible for applying the rules appropriately in the case of procedures in clinical trials. Fiscal intermediaries and carriers audit these interpretations by providers in clinical trials, as they now audit bills from providers for care outside of clinical trials. Advice or an interpretation could, of course, be requested of HCFA at any time. In addition, HCFA would retain the right to initiate its own review, without being asked, if it believes there is an issue to be explored, to carry out a random check, or for another reason.

The committee recognizes that creating definitions that neatly separate "category A" and "category B" procedures will not be simple, and disagreements are inescapable about where the line between "A" and "B" should be drawn in specific cases. Table 3-1 gives a few examples of how the definitions might work.

Wherever the separation lies, some procedures will fall into a "gray zone." HCFA can narrow the gray zone by applying the definitions to a wide range of real and hypothetical procedures, and stating whether the procedures would or would not be eligible for reimbursement. To deal with cases in which uncertainty remains, HCFA should set up a process to rule quickly on reimbursement eligibility. With accumulated experience, the number of gray zone cases should decline, as has been the case with FDA classification of devices into categories A and B.

TABLE 3-1. Reimbursement Eligibility for Procedures Under Recommendation 2

Standard Procedure and Indication	Innovation and/or Indication	Circumstances of Trial, Nature of Innovation	Reimbursement Eligibility: Yes/No/HCFA Review
Open cholecystectomy	Laparoscopic cholecystectomy	If neither this nor other "keyhole surgeries" were being reimbursed by HCFA, this would be considered a major departure from standard practice	No
Open cholecystectomy	Laparoscopic cholecystectomy	If other "keyhole surgeries" were already being reimbursed by HCFA, this would fall in the "gray zone"	HCFA review?
Mastectomy for early breast cancer	Lumpectomy for early breast cancer	Lumpectomy is a variation on mastectomy	Yes
Standard surgery for parathyroid disease: removal of some parathyroid glands with confirmation by pathology during surgery	Surgery for parathyroid disease with physiologic calcium measurement to determine surgical endpoint	The procedure is the same; only monitoring is different	Yes
Optic nerve decompression surgery (ONDS) for pseudotumor cerebrii	ONDS for nonarteritic ischemic optic neuropathy	New indication for standard procedure, but had been used and reimbursed for new indication outside of trial	Yes (this would qualify under recommendation 1, because Medicare had been paying for patients outside of trials)

Open CABG	Midline CABG (minimally invasive procedure)	Could be considered next-generation open CABG	Yes or gray zone
Human liver transplant	Pig liver transplant	Used only in experimental situations; significantly different from standard intervention	No
Heart transplant or aggressive medical treatment for congestive heart failure	Battista procedure: removal of damaged cardiac tissue	Completely new procedure.	No
Pharmacologic or no treatment	Fetal cell transplant for Parkinson's disease	Completely new procedure	No

NOTE: Procedures in the table are for illustration only and are treated as though they were new in 1999 and relevant to the Medicare population, even though that is not the case for all examples. In each instance, the judgment about reimbursement eligibility is made assuming that the trial was taking place before HCFA had begun "legitimate reimbursement" for the procedure for the specified indication. By "legitimate reimbursement," we mean that reimbursement was made for claims that disclosed the nature of the procedure and the indication for which it was performed.

In this table, "HCFA review" means that the procedure falls in the "gray zone" (or for some other reason, the principal investigator is uncertain about reimbursement eligibility), and a determination of eligibility could be made by HCFA.

If a trial is initiated after reimbursement has become standard practice, the "fundamental" rule—that procedures that are covered in the course of usual medical practice would also be covered in clinical trials—would apply, and reimbursement would be allowed. For any procedure not eligible for reimbursement under the stated rule, investigators could apply to HCFA for reimbursement as an exception.

The committee has not attempted to specify an institutional mechanism under which HCFA might carry out the tasks required by this recommendation. However, the committee notes that the new Medicare Coverage Advisory Committee* might provide the needed expertise for the task of defining categories A and B and ruling quickly on "gray zone" cases that arise.

RECOMMENDATION 3. For claims submitted in accordance with both the fundamental recommendation (No. 1) and the special recommendation for procedures (No. 2), no special precertification by HCFA, or any other administrative process, should be required of clinical trial researchers or providers participating in trials before they submit claims for reimburseable services. Claims should be submitted in the same way they are for treatment outside of trials.

Practitioners and institutions would be expected to submit reimbursement claims for services to patients in clinical trials under rules outlined in recommendations 1 and 2. With a clear statement of reimbursement policy, such claims should pose difficulties no different from those arising in the administration of coverage and reimbursement rules for claims for care outside of trials.

Investigators and providers would not be routinely required to submit documentation about the trial to HCFA, but HCFA could, at any time, request such documentation to confirm that the clinical trial meets current standards for scientific merit and has the relevant IRB approval.

RECOMMENDATION 4. If Medicare or trial sponsors fail to cover clinical care costs, patients should not be billed for those costs above what they would pay if they were not in a trial.

This recommendation is not one that can be enforced as part of a reimbursement policy by HCFA; however, the committee believes it is an important principle that could be adopted by clinical trial sponsors and investigators. It also could be incorporated in any legislation passed to implement the committee's recommendations.

RECOMMENDATION 5. Medicare members of managed care plans should have the same reimbursement eligibility for care in clinical trials as those enrolled in fee-for-service Medicare, but not beyond the limits of the managed care contract.

---

*The Medicare Coverage Advisory Committee (MCAC) was established by HCFA to provide guidance on coverage issues. The 120-member committee will function through specialty panels of not more than 15 members each. The MCAC had its first meeting in September 1999.

Nearly one Medicare beneficiary in five belongs to a capitated plan—an HMO or some other form of managed care. That number is likely to increase over time. It is vital, therefore, that the committee's recommendations carry over to patients served outside traditional Medicare. Managed care plans must provide all benefits offered under traditional Medicare. (Most offer additional benefits, including coverage of outpatient drugs.) Accordingly, the committee recommends that managed care plans be required to offer Medicare beneficiaries access to clinical trials involving services available within their networks. If, for example, a plan routinely covers a particular drug, it should cover it in a trial, as well. If the plan limits the choice of drugs to those listed on a formulary, the plan should not be required to cover a nonformulary drug in a trial.

Under point-of-service plans, patients should have the right to go outside the managed care network to participate in a trial, under the terms stipulated in the plan for point-of-service care, but no such right should be inferred under plans that limit enrollees to the plan's providers. This recommendation is not comprehensive, but is suggestive of a policy for managed care. Full implementation will require additional thought when HCFA adopts a clinical trial reimbursement policy, but the committee urges that the new policy not create obstacles to clinical trial enrollment for beneficiaries in managed care.

RECOMMENDATION 6. In addition to providing routine coverage through the proposed policy, the committee urges HCFA to use its existing authority to support selected trials and to assist in the development of new trials. In selected clinical trials, the committee believes that HCFA should do more than pay for routine patient care according to the recommendations already stated. Medicare should (1) provide additional reimbursement in a limited number of trials and (2) identify emerging or current methods of care of particular importance to the Medicare population and work with other organizations to initiate trials.

Researchers should be able to apply to HCFA for reimbursement above routine rates in cases meriting special treatment. Such trials could include some interventions that do not qualify under the basic recommendations, such as "category A" procedures, primary and secondary screening, diagnostics, and interventions not usually covered by Medicare (e.g., behavioral interventions). The rationale for extending coverage is straightforward. HCFA has a large stake in determining whether more effective or less costly alternatives to current interventions may exist, preventing ineffective procedures from becoming common practice, and facilitating the identification of innovations that would benefit the Medicare population.

For example, a behavioral intervention, which normally would not be covered, might replace a more expensive drug or surgical intervention to the benefit of both patients' health and Medicare finances. HCFA should have sole authority to decide whether to extend coverage and should make such determinations expeditiously. The committee assumes that only a few trials would be appropriate for such exceptional treatment each year.

In the case of interventions of particular importance to the Medicare population, HCFA should collaborate with the National Institutes of Health (NIH) or others to see that appropriate trials are fielded. HCFA should cover routine patient care costs for these trials along the lines of the committee's basic recommendation. It could also fund other costs as well, under the exceptions procedure described in the preceding paragraph. But the objective is to encourage trials, not necessarily to pay for them. Such an active role would not be new for HCFA. This recommendation follows the model of the ongoing study of lung volume reduction surgery, which grew out of collaboration among HCFA, NIH, and the Agency for Health Care Policy and Research (AHCPR), at HCFA's initiative.

RECOMMENDATION 7. Every trial for which some Medicare reimbursement is sought should be entered into a national registry of clinical trials.

Reimbursement claims should bear an identification number assigned by the registry. A registry will facilitate ex post audits of reimbursement claims, HCFA's main tool for monitoring clinical trial coverage and detecting potential abuse. But identification of a claim as part of a clinical trial should not be relevant to the reimbursement decision.

The committee recognizes that implementation of this recommendation will necessarily take some time. Therefore, the committee's recommendations regarding reimbursement of routine patient care costs do not hinge on the existence of a clinical trials registry. Until a registry is in operation, reimbursement claims for interventions associated with a clinical trial should be denoted on the form, in a manner HCFA specifies. However, a registry would contribute to uniform administration and permit HCFA and others to carry out analyses of clinical trials and the costs of implementing the recommendations put forward here. It should, therefore, be put in place as quickly as possible.

Ideally, such a registry should include all publicly and privately sponsored trials before they begin accruing patients, thereby providing a link to all claims for Medicare patients in clinical trials. If the goal of creating such a registry is accepted, the practical question of how best to achieve it must be addressed. It would be possible to build upon the registry currently under development at NIH by broadening the definition of trials to be included and consulting widely on how to present data. Or a separate registry could be created.

Whether the registry should operate within NIH or elsewhere merits consideration. The design of the NIH registry has been underway for some time. Its designers claim that it will be functioning, at least in part, by early 2000. Redirecting any ongoing effort will be difficult for reasons that are well understood. If it were concluded that converting this limited registry into an inclusive national registry would be needlessly cumbersome, the creation of a separate comprehensive registry, serving objectives beyond those of NIH, or even of HCFA, should be explored. The committee urges the Secretary of HHS to examine this issue promptly, set a timetable for completion of a registry, and seek adequate funding for it.

ADMINISTRATIVE AND COST IMPLICATIONS

Implementation of the committee's recommendations would likely cause some increase in administrative costs to HCFA. In making its recommendations, the committee strove to minimize potential administrative burdens. It is the committee's judgment that any added administrative costs required by institution of this reimbursement policy will be small.

Effects of the committee's recommendations on benefit costs are more important and far more uncertain. For several reasons, the cost impact of these recommendations is likely to be quite small. First, the recommended reimbursement policy is designed to limit payments for an individual to roughly the cost of "standard care" for which he or she would be eligible if not enrolled in the trial. This limitation does not imply that each individual would have chosen standard care that cost the same as the care in the clinical trial, so in individual cases, the cost of actual care in the trial might be higher or lower than forgone care outside the trial. Although the incremental cost of routine care in clinical trials is not known with certainty, it is almost surely small in comparison to the costs otherwise incurred by Medicare. Some clinical trial groups claim that the costs of treating patients in some trials may be less than treating them outside of trials. Second, clinical trials hold the long-term prospect of identifying ineffective interventions, which would fall out of favor in the clinical community, or could be excluded from coverage, in some cases saving Medicare dollars.

Finally, only a tiny fraction of Medicare patients participate in clinical trials. No accurate count of clinical trial participants at any point in time exists, but the Lewin Group has estimated that about 265,000 people in the United States participate in clinical trials each year, including about 161,000 Medicare beneficiaries—less than 0.5 percent of the 38 million Medicare enrollees in 1997 (Dobson and Sturm, 1999). Clearly, the proportion of Medicare beneficiaries in clinical trials is quite small. The available evidence suggests that Medicare already pays for a large proportion of routine patient care in such trials, including both costs for which no reimbursement is sought, and claims that are submitted and rejected.

The largest effect on Medicare costs could come from the speedier determination of the efficacy of innovative or experimental procedures, drugs, and devices. Some will be cost increasing. Others will be cost reducing. Whether the net effect is to raise or lower total Medicare spending, the speedy determination of what works and what does not work will benefit the Medicare population and the nation as a whole.

CONCLUSION

Clinical trials are integral to modern medical care and to the progress of medical science. Although HCFA has issued little explicit policy about payment for routine patient care for patients in clinical trials, the Medicare statute has been widely interpreted to exclude reimbursement for such care. However, evidence is ample to suggest that providers submit claims for routine care for Medicare beneficiaries in trials without noting the existence of the clinical trial, and HCFA's financial contractors usually pay them. The thrust of the committee's recommendations is that nothing should be done that would materially curtail Medicare's reimbursement for routine patient care costs for patients in clinical trials. On the contrary, HCFA should encourage such trials and even extend reimbursement in a limited number of specifically approved exceptional cases. To achieve these goals, the committee believes that HCFA should assure patients in clinical trials the same reimbursement of routine patient care that is available to patients who are not in trials. Extending reimbursement to certain procedures that represent modifications of current practice and distinguishing those from procedures for which risks and benefits are largely unknown will require some additional effort by HCFA, but it is an essential component of the committee's recommendations. The fundamental recommendation—reimbursement independent of trial participation—should be implemented relatively easily.

References

American Association of Health Plans. AAHP Board of Directors Agreement Between AAHP and NIH for Support of Clinical Trials. Dated December 11, 1998. [http://www.aahp.org/menus/index.cfm?CFID=84873&CFTOKEN=5124]

Ault, T., Director, Bureau of Policy Development, Health Care Financing Administration. 1996. Statement on Investigational Medical Devices, Committee on Governmental Affairs, Permanent Subcommittee on Investigations, U.S. Senate, February 14, 1996.

Barlow, W., S. Taplin, D. Seger, J. Beckord, L. Ichikawa. 1998. Medical Care Costs of Cancer Patients on Protocol. NCI Meeting, Bethesda, MD: July 7.

Bull, J. P. 1959. The historical development of clinical therapeutic trials. *J Chronic Dis* 10:218–48.

Cochrane Library Controlled Trials Register. 1999. In: *The Cochrane Library* [database on CD-ROM]. Oxford, England: Update Software, issue 2.

DeParle, N.-A.M., Administrator, Health Care Financing Administration. 1998. Statement on Health Technology Assessment, Labor and Human Resources Committee, Subcommittee on Public Health and Safety, U.S. Senate, March 12, 1998.

Department of Defense 1999. DoD/NCI agreement expands TRICARE benefit to include cancer prevention trials. DoD Worldwide web site. [tricare.osd.mil/main/news/art0706.html]

Department of Defense/National Cancer Institute. 1996. Interagency Agreement Between the Department of Defense and National Cancer Institute for Partnership in Clinical Trials for Cancer.

Department of Veterans Affairs. Worldwide web site, August 1999.

Department of Veterans Affairs/National Cancer Institute. 1997. Interagency Agreement Between the Department of Veterans Affairs and the National Cancer Institute for a Partnership in Clinical Trials for Cancer.

Dickersin, K., and Y.I. Min. 1993. Publication bias: The problem that won't go away. *Ann N Y Acad Sci* 703:135–46.

Dobson, A., and Sturm, E. 1999. Reimbursement of Routine Patient Care Costs in Clinical Trials. (Report to the Institute of Medicine Committee on Routine Patient Care

Costs in Clinical Trials for Medicare Beneficiaries.) The Lewin Group, Fairfax, Va., 1999.

Doll, R. 1982. Clinical trials: Retrospect and prospect. *Stat Med* 1:337–44.

Evans, R. 1992. Public and private insurer designation of transplantation programs. *Transplantation* 53(5):1041–6.

Fireman, B., L. Fehrenbacher, L. Gruskin, and T. Ray. 1998. The Cost of Care in Cancer Clinical Trials at Kaiser Permanente, Northern California. NCI Meeting, Bethesda MD: July 7.

Fisher, R. A. 1926. The arrangement of field experiments. *J Ministry Agricult Gt Brit* 33:503–13.

Fisher, R. A. 1935. *The Design of Experiments*. Edinburgh: Oliver and Boyd.

Hartwig, J. E. 1996. Medical Coverage of Investigational Devices. Testimony Before the Committee on Governmental Affairs, Permanent Subcommittee on Investigations, U.S. Senate, February 14, 1996.

Health Care Financing Administration/Food and Drug Administration. 1995. Interagency Agreement Between the Food and Drug Administration and the Health Care Financing Administration Regarding Medicare Coverage of Certain Investigational Medical Devices (IDE Memorandum D95-2). Photocopy.

Hennekens, C. H., and J. E. Buring. 1987. *Epidemiology in Medicine*. Boston: Little, Brown, and Co.

Holohan, T. V., and H. Handelsman. 1996. Lung-volume reduction surgery for end-stage chronic obstructive pulmonary disease. *Health Technol Assess (Rockv)* 10(Sept.):1–30.

Lilienfeld, A. M. 1982. Ceteris paribus: The evolution of the clinical trial. *Bull Hist Med* 56: 1–18.

McCray, A. National Library of Medicine, NIH. 1999. Personal communication to H. Gelband.

Medical Research Council. 1948. Streptomycin treatment of pulmonary tuberculosis. *BMJ* 2:769–82.

Meinert, C. L. 1986. *Clinical Trials: Design, Conduct, and Analysis*. Oxford: Oxford University Press, pp. 3–10.

Newcomer, L. 1999. Medical Director, United Health Group, personal communication, August 1999.

O'Rourke, P. 1999. Office of the Director, NIH. Personal communication to Hellen Gelband.

Szymanski, J. 1999. Office of the Assistant Secretary of Defense (Health Affairs), personal communication, October 1999.

U.S. General Accounting Office. 1997. Cancer Clinical Trials: Medicare Reimbursement Denials (GAO/HEHS-98-15R). Washington, D.C.: GAO.

U.S. General Accounting Office. 1999. NIH Clinical Trials: Various Factors Affect Patient Participation (GAO/HEHS-99-182). Washington, D.C.: GAO.

Wagner, J. L., S. R. Alberts, J. A. Sloan, S. Cha, J. Killian, M. J. O'Connell et al. 1999. Incremental costs of enrolling cancer patients in clinical trials: A population-based study. *J Natl Cancer Inst* 91(10):847–53.

Zelen, M. 1993. Large simple trials. In *Clinical Trials and Statistics: Proceedings of a Symposium*. Washington, D.C.: National Academy Press.

APPENDIX A

Glossary, Acronyms, and Abbreviations

GLOSSARY

blinding (synonym: masking) Keeping secret group assignment (e.g., to treatment or control) from the study participants or investigators. Blinding is used to protect against the possibility that knowledge of assignment may affect patient response to treatment, provider behaviors (performance bias), or outcome assessment (detection bias). Blinding is not always practical (e.g., when comparing surgery to drug treatment). The importance of blinding depends on how objective the outcome measure is; blinding is more important for less easily measurable and quantifiable outcome measures such as pain or quality of life.

carriers Private insurance companies that process Medicare Part B claims under contract to HCFA. They apply the Medicare coverage rules to determine the appropriateness of claims and issue payments to providers for the government.

clinical trial A formal study carried out according to a prospectively defined protocol that is intended to discover or verify the safety and effectiveness in human beings of interventions to promote well-being, or to prevent, diagnose, or treat illness. The term may refer to a controlled or uncontrolled trial. In a strict sense, the modifier "clinical" could be reserved for trials carried out in a clinical setting involving clinical disease, but in practice, its use has been extended to include other types of trials, such as health promotion and disease prevention, and trials carried out in the community. "Trials," without a modifier, is used synonymously with "clinical trials" in this report.

diagnosis-related group (DRG) A set of related diagnoses, generally requiring similar treatment and length of stay for necessary procedures, used as

67

the basis for inpatient payment under the Medicare prospective payment system (PPS).

effectiveness   Effectiveness describes the extent to which a specific intervention, when used under *ordinary* circumstances, does what it is intended to do. Effectiveness, therefore, takes into account the fact that, in any group of individuals, some will not take the intervention as prescribed, or will take other actions that may compromise the effect of the intervention (e.g., take drugs that might interact with the test intervention).

efficacy   Efficacy is defined as the extent to which an intervention produces a beneficial result under *ideal* conditions.

end-stage renal disease (ESRD)   Irreversible kidney failure. To survive, the patient must either receive a kidney transplant or periodic kidney dialysis. Individuals with ESRD are eligible for Medicare benefits.

fiscal intermediaries (FI)   Private insurance companies that process Medicare Part A claims under contract to HCFA. They apply the Medicare coverage rules to determine the appropriateness of claims and issue payments to providers for the government.

HCFA   The Health Care Financing Administration, an agency within the U.S. Department of Health and Human Services that administers the Medicare and Medicaid programs.

institutional review board (IRB)   A committee or board associated with a specific institution, constituted according to rules set by the U.S. Department of Health and Human Services, responsible for reviewing, approving, and monitoring research studies involving human beings to be carried out in that institution. Review focuses mainly on the ethics of the proposed research, the informed consent process, and other issues related to study participants.

intention-to-treat (analysis)   An intention-to-treat analysis is one in which outcomes for all the participants in a trial are analyzed according to the intervention to which they were allocated, whether they received it or not. Intention-to-treat analyses mirror the noncompliance and treatment changes that are likely to occur when the intervention is used in practice, and eliminate the potential effect introducing attrition bias by excluding some participants from the analysis.

Investigational Device Exemption (IDE)   An exemption given by the FDA to the manufacturer of a new medical device or to an independent investigator permitting evaluation of the device in human beings in specified studies under specified conditions. The studies are intended to produce information required for approval of the device for marketing.

Investigational New Drug Exemption (IND)   An exemption given by the FDA to the manufacturer of a new drug or to an independent investigator permitting evaluation of the drug in human beings in specified studies under specified conditions. In some cases, INDs may also be needed to allow study of already-approved drugs for new ("unlabelled") indications. The studies are intended to produce information required for approval of the device for marketing.

managed care plan   A general term applied to a wide range of insurance plans, including HMOs, where choice of providers is limited and administrative measures control utilization of services. The types of Medicare managed care plans include health maintenance organizations (HMOs), competitive medical plans (CMPs), and health care prepayment plans (HCPPs). The Balanced Budget Act of 1997 expands the types of managed care plans that can participate in Medicare.

medical device   Diagnostic or therapeutic equipment that does not interact chemically with a person's body. Includes, for example, diagnostic tests, kits, pacemakers and other heart rhythm devices, arterial grafts, stents, intraocular lenses, and artificial heart valves and joints.

meta-analysis   The use of statistical techniques in a systematic review to integrate the results of the included studies. Also used to refer to systematic reviews that use meta-analysis.

PDQ   The Physician Data Query system of the National Cancer Institute, which consists of a registry of most NCI-sponsored clinical trials as well as some other trials (industry-sponsored, foreign-sponsored). Other components of PDQ are site- and stage-specific descriptions of cancers and state-of-the-art treatment options. PDQ is accessible to the public as well as physicians, via internet or telephone requests.

phases of trials   Clinical trials are classified by phase most commonly for drugs, biologics, and devices in the FDA approval process for marketing (although the trials themselves may extend beyond the date of approval). NIH also describes trials by phase, for example, trials in cancer and AIDS, which are listed in their respective registries by phase. Clear lines do not necessarily demarcate one phase from another, however, and trials may be denoted as "phase 1/2" or "phase 3/4." In trials undertaken other than for marketing approval, a trial designated as phase 2 or 3 does not necessarily imply the completion of earlier phases: a phase 3 trial may be the first undertaken for a specific intervention.

phase 1 trial   First studies in people, to evaluate chemical action, appropriate dosage, and safety. Usually enrolls small numbers of participants and typically has no comparison group.

phase 2 trial   Provides preliminary information about how well the new drug works and generates more information about safety and benefit. Usually includes comparison group; patients may be assigned to groups by randomization.

phase 3 trial   Compares intervention with the current standard or placebo to assess dosage effects, effectiveness, and safety. Almost always uses random allocation to assign treatment. Typically involves many people (hundreds or thousands) but may be smaller.

phase 4 trial   Compares intervention with control intervention (with assignment to groups by randomization or some other scheme) with long-term follow-up focusing on specific clinical events related to safety and efficacy. For drugs, phase 4 trials may be required by FDA after approval for marketing has been granted.

placebo   An inactive substance or procedure administered to a patient, usually to compare its effects with those of a real drug or other intervention, but sometimes for the psychological benefit to the patient through a belief that s/he is receiving treatment. Placebos are used in clinical trials to blind people to their treatment allocation. Placebos should be indistinguishable from the active intervention to ensure adequate blinding.

principal investigator (PI)   The individual responsible for directing a research project.

protocol-induced costs   Patient care costs incurred in a clinical trial for services necessary solely to satisfy data collection needs of the clinical trial, such as monthly CT scans for a condition usually requiring only a single scan. Care that would be required under standard treatment—even if it also is required by the trial protocol—would *not* be considered protocol-induced.

randomization (random assignment)   A method that uses the play of chance to assign participants to comparison groups in a trial, by using a random numbers table or a computer-generated random sequence. Random allocation implies that each individual or unit being entered into a trial has the same chance of receiving each of the possible interventions. It also implies that the probability that an individual will receive a particular intervention is independent of the probability that any other individual will receive the same intervention.

routine patient care   Care that would be received by a patient undergoing "standard treatment." This would include such items as room and board for patients who are hospitalized, diagnostic and laboratory tests and monitoring appropriate to the patient's condition, post-surgical care when indicated, office visits, and so on.

standard treatment   An accepted mode of treatment for a given condition.

ACRONYMS AND ABBREVIATIONS

AAHP   American Association of Health Plans
AHCPR   Agency for Health Care Policy and Research
AMC   Academic Medical Center

ASCO	American Society of Clinical Oncology
CDC	Centers for Disease Control and Prevention
CFR	Code of Federal Regulations
CMP	competitive medical plan
CT	computerized tomography
DHHS	Department of Health and Human Services
DoD	Department of Defense
DRG	diagnosis-related group
FDA	Food and Drug Administration
GAO	General Accounting Office
GCRC	General Clinical Research Center
GHC	Group Health Cooperative of Puget Sound
HCFA	Health Care Financing Administration
HCPP	health care prepayment plan
HHA	Home Health Agency
HMO	health maintenance organization
IDE	Investigational Device Exemption
IND	Investigational New Drug Exemption
IOM	Institute of Medicine
IRB	institutional review board
KPNC	Kaiser Permanente of Northern California
LVRS	lung volume reduction surgery
MRA	magnetic resonance angiography
NCI	National Cancer Institute
NHLBI	National Heart, Lung and Blood Institute
NIDDK	National Institute of Diabetes and Digestive and Kidney Diseases
NIH	National Institutes of Health
NLM	National Library of Medicine
OIG	Office of the Inspector General
ONDS	optic nerve decompression surgery
OPRR	Office of Protection from Research Risks
PDQ	Physician Data Query
PET	positron-emission tomography
PI	principal investigator

PPS   prospective payment system
PRO   Peer Review Organization
ProPAC   Prospective Payment Assessment Commission
PTCA   percutaneous transluminal coronary angioplasty

SNF   skilled nursing facility
SPN   solitary pulmonary nodule

VA   Department of Veterans Affairs

APPENDIX B

Committee Biographies

HENRY J. AARON, Ph.D. (*Chair*), is a Senior Fellow in economic studies at the Brookings Institution. He is currently chair of the board of the National Academy of Social Insurance, president of the Association of Public Policy and Management, and a member and councilor of the American Academy of Arts and Sciences. He was an Assistant Secretary for Planning and Evaluation in the Department of Health, Education, and Welfare during the Carter administration, and is a former chairman of the Advisory Council on Social Security. He has written extensively on financial aspects of the U.S. health care system, including Medicare.

ROBERT M. CALIFF, M.D., is Professor of Medicine in the Division of Cardiology at Duke University Medical Center. He also holds the following titles: Associate Vice Chancellor for Clinical Research and Director of the Duke Clinical Research Institute, as well as editor-in-chief of the *American Heart Journal.* He has been a principal investigator for some of the largest recent U.S.-based cardiology trials, including CAVEAT (Coronary Angioplasty Versus Excisional Atherectomy Trial), GUSTO (Global Utilization of Streptokinase and t-PA for Occluded Coronary Arteries), EPIC (Evaluation of c7E3 Fab for the Prevention of Ischemic Complications), and TAMI (Thrombolysis and Angioplasty in Myocardial Infarction). He has written extensively about clinical and economic outcomes in ischemic heart disease. Dr. Califf was also on the 1969 AAAA South Carolina Championship Basketball team.

KAY DICKERSIN, Ph.D., Associate Professor, Department of Community Health, Brown University School of Medicine, is co-director of the New England Cochrane Center. Her primary academic interests are evidence-based medicine, clinical trial design, and meta-analysis. Dr. Dickersin directs the coordinating center for two federally funded, multicenter randomized trials: The Ischemic Optic Decompression Trial and the Surgical Treatments Outcomes Project for Dysfunctional Uterine Bleeding.

BERTIE A. FORD, M.S., R.N., O.C.N., is a clinical nurse specialist with Amgen. Until taking up this position, she had been Manager of Clinical Research and the Cancer Registry at Grant/Riverside Hospitals, Columbus, Ohio, since February 1998. Earlier, Ms. Ford was Clinical Trials Program Coordinator in the Ohio State University Department of Internal Medicine for most of the period from 1988. During that period she spent a brief time at Pharmacia in clinical research, and earlier, she held various positions with oncology research groups. She has recently been appointed to the steering council of the Oncology Nursing Society and wrote several chapters for the society's clinical trial manual for nurses. She is currently president of the Columbus Chapter of the National Black Nurses Association. Ms. Ford served on the National Cancer Policy Board from 1997 through April 1999.

PETER D. FOX, Ph.D., has been an independent consultant specializing in managed care since 1991. For the 10 previous years he was a vice president at Lewin and Associates (now The Lewin Group), a consulting company. His clients include managed care organizations, health care provider groups, employers, Taft-Hartley trust funds, government agencies, and foundations. He previously held positions in the federal government, including serving as Director of the Office of Policy Analysis in the Health Care Financing Administration. He has written three books and many articles and book chapters on issues related to health care financing and delivery with an emphasis on managed care.

LANCE LIEBMAN, L.L.B., William S. Beinecke Professor of Law, Columbia University Law School, is Director of Columbia's Parker School of Foreign and Comparative Law and Director of the American Law Institute. He has had a distinguished career in public service and academic law over the past 30 years. From 1991 to 1996, he was Dean of the Columbia University Law School.

JOHN M. LUDDEN, M.D., is Associate Clinical Professor, Department of Ambulatory Care and Prevention, Harvard Medical School. Previously, Dr. Ludden was Senior Vice President, Medical Affairs of Harvard Pilgrim Health Care, where he headed the Department of Medical Affairs and Health Policy from 1994 to 1998. Dr. Ludden served as Corporate Medical Director from 1983 to 1994. He joined Harvard Community Health Plan in 1972, where he was a staff psychiatrist and Director of the Kenmore Health Center. Before joining Harvard Community Health Plan, Dr. Ludden served as Director and Co-Director of the Alcohol Clinic at the Peter Bent Brigham Hospital in Boston. He was also Chief of the Psychiatric Division of the Directorate of Mental Hygiene at the U.S. Disciplinary Barracks in Ft. Leavenworth, Kansas, and psychiatrist in the U.S. Army. Dr. Ludden serves on the boards of the National Committee for

Quality Assurance and the American College of Physician Executives. Dr. Ludden is certified in Psychiatry by the American Board of Psychiatry and Neurology and in Medical Management by the American Board of Medical Management. Dr. Ludden completed his psychiatric residency at the Massachusetts Mental Health Center. He received a B.A. from Harvard College and an M.D. from Harvard Medical School. He completed the program for Management Development at the Harvard Graduate School of Business.

ROBERT S. McDONOUGH, M.D., J.D., M.P.P, is Medical Director and Senior Consultant in the Clinical Policy Unit of Aetna U.S. Healthcare. He is responsible for developing clinical policies and clinical guidelines that apply to all of Aetna U.S. Healthcare's products (indemnity, PPO, POS, and HMO plans), and for the preventive services guidelines and policies, continuing medical education programs for physicians, and pharmacy formulary evaluations.

WILLIAM T. McGIVNEY, Ph.D., has been Chief Executive Officer of the National Comprehensive Cancer Network—an association of the major cancer research centers in the United States—since 1997. In earlier positions, he was vice president for clinical and coverage policy for Aetna Health Plans (and also held other positions with Aetna) and director of the Division of Health Care Technology for the American Medical Association.

ROSEMARY ROSSO, J.D., is a breast cancer survivor and a member of the Metropolitan Washington Breast Cancer Coalition and the National Breast Cancer Coalition. Through these organizations, she has worked to encourage greater access to and participation in clinical trials for breast cancer research. Ms. Rosso also holds other local and national cancer patient and advocacy positions, including member of the U.S. Department of Defense Breast Cancer Research Program's Integration Panel. Ms. Rosso is a senior attorney with the Federal Trade Commission.

ELIZABETH STONER, M.D., is Vice President for Clinical Research, Endocrine/Metabolism and Contract and Cost Management at Merck. She is responsible for the financing and budgets of clinical trials, including those performed by contract research organizations.

BOB THOMPSON, M.S., M.A., Senior Manager, Reimbursement and Economics Department, Medtronic, works in the areas of strategic reimbursement planning, health outcomes, and cost-effectiveness research. He also worked in Medtronic's Neurological Division for 5 years, in the same three areas, as well as in clinical practice guidelines and health outcomes software development. As part of his responsibilities, Mr. Thompson has worked with Medicare and other payers for the past 7 years.

PETER J. WHITEHOUSE, M.D., Ph.D., is Professor in the Department of Neurology, Psychiatry, Neuroscience, and Biomedical Ethics at Case Western Reserve University School of Medicine. His research focuses on the basic and clinical neuroscience of aging-related diseases, particularly Alzheimer's disease. He has extensive experience in drug trials for Alzheimer's disease, with a special interest in quality of life measurement, bioethics, and geriatric care systems. He has served as a consultant and advisor to numerous national and international professional, government, and private organizations.